The Quest for

PEACE,

LOVE,

and a
24" WAIST

The Quest for
PEACE,
LOVE,
and a
24" WAIST

DEBORAH LOW

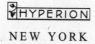

NEW YORK

Copyright © 2002, 2004 Deborah Low
Previously published by Bonneville Books.

Library of Congress Cataloging-in-Publication Data

Low, Deborah
    The quest for peace, love, and a 24" waist / by Deborah Low.
        p.   cm.
    Previously published: Utah : Bonneville Books, 2002.
    Includes bibliographical references.
    ISBN: 0-7868-8888-1
    1. Weight loss—Psychological aspects.   2. Body image.   I. Title.

    RM222.2.L673 2004
    613.7—dc21

                                                    2003056633

Hyperion books are available for special promotions and premiums. For details contact Michael Rentas, Manager, Inventory and Premium Sales, Hyperion, 77 West 66th Street, 11th floor, New York, New York 10023-6298, or call 212-456-0133.

FIRST EDITION

10 9 8 7 6 5 4 3 2 1

To my mother and father

who, in their own individual ways,
taught me that love is all we have.

CONTENTS

ACKNOWLEDGMENTS

Thanks . . .

to the hundreds of men and women over the years whom I have had the pleasure to train and counsel. You have risked sharing your personal struggles with me. Your honesty and hard work has been a gift. Thanks for letting me see you sweat!

to my editor, Mary Ellen O'Neill, for believing in my message and making my transition to Hyperion so seamless.

to my talented brother, Warren. You never cease to inspire me.

to Dean and Justice, my secret happiness recipe.

to Jude Hedlund for welcoming me into Deepak Chopra's ever-inspiring Center for Well Being, and allowing me to give a little back.

to all of those who have gone before me with the pure intention to inspire, share, heal, and love others.

Without you, this book would not exist.

You cannot teach a man anything;
you can only help him find it within himself.

—*Galileo*

In Search of the Grail

WHEN IT COMES to body image and dieting, my story is similar to that of millions of other women around the world. For many of us, what begins as an innocent-enough plan soon morphs into an all-consuming quest for the culturally based, female version of the Holy Grail: Peace, Love, and a 24" Waist—not necessarily in that order.

Originally, we only wanted to lose weight, yet somewhere along the path we began to equate happiness with the size of our waists. Where did we take a wrong turn?

Each one of us has a story to tell, but our reasons vary as to why we've let the judgment of our bodies distract us from the peace, love, and happiness to which we are entitled. We are all navigating through a universal tale, looking for *the* moral to our stories. Regardless of our differences, we all want to be free from the chains of restrictive diets and punishing beliefs that we hold about ourselves.

As a personal trainer, I have worked with hundreds of men and women over the last decade. People come to me for a myriad of reasons, yet wanting to lose weight is still their number one motivation. For these particular clients, it's still overwhelming to discover how many of them are unhappy in life, believing that excess weight is the source from which all other problems stem. Millions of women deny themselves happiness, believing that they will *only* be satisfied with their lives when they lose weight. By empowering this belief, they have already sacrificed who they are to the number on the scale.

Most weight-loss quests begin with an incomplete map, namely, a restrictive diet. Every day, dieters get lost down this narrow path and the likelihood of experiencing permanent life-enriching weight loss is no more probable than developing "washboard" abdominal muscles without doing a single sit-up. Yet, when we expand our attention and focus on the soul's desire, an amazing thing happens. Joy and happiness return, and our energies are directed toward fulfilling our dreams and passions. In our soul's plan for us, there is no deprivation or self-judgment. In fact, we finally understand that we are not searching to find freedom in a diet or exercise plan; but instead, we are looking to find tools that help us tap into our own sources of *intrinsic* motivation. *Intrinsic* simply refers to the essential nature of *who we are.*

Through greater self-awareness, all of our desires can be realized, including weight loss. When the focus is expanded to see the *whole* picture, the emotional battle with food ends. It is simply food, and an excess of physical and mental weight that we no longer choose to carry throughout life.

With my clients and myself, I no longer focus on waistlines but instead on the gifts that healthy living brings to our mind, body, and spirit. *Inspired* means to be *in spirit,* which is the intangible measurement of any health and fitness accomplishment. Losing weight is a legitimate health goal; losing your spirit along with the pounds is not. Our job on this earth is not to get thin, then to start living, but instead to hold the highest concept of ourselves in every moment. When you make this your job, your body will mend itself. You will finally be feeding your soul.

This book is about successfully losing weight—but regardless of the size of your body, the message throughout is universal, aimed to empower the spirit of anyone—dieter and non-dieter alike. Use this information to help you remember that experiencing peace, love, and happiness in our lives starts with a simple shift in our awareness, available to us whenever we choose. This book will lead you through the information, questions, and exercises needed for you to make this shift, and in doing so, help you to end the struggle with your body and lose weight with joy.

Your journey through this book will be divided into stages. Suspend your doubts and embark on this adventure—

open to the possibility that weight loss is about gaining health and experiencing joy. Your quest will unfold as follows:

- Challenging beliefs—why are you on this weight-loss quest?

- Avoiding ego threats—learning to see the *self* in a new light.

- Discovering your intrinsic motivators—the ultimate tool for realigning with your essential nature.

- Soul food—for a *whole* life.

- Exploring the splendid world of food.

- Exercising your right to enjoyment—a new set of guidelines for being active.

- Conscious living—priceless tools for a well-planned quest.

- Creating a masterpiece—putting it all together.

Let's begin.

CHAPTER ONE

I Am a House—My Own Quest

I AM A WOMAN; and like you, I have been blessed with the gift of owning my own body (or renting one, at least, for those who have not ruled out the notion of reincarnation). Yet in the many years that I've lived in this house I must admit that I've been a difficult tenant.

I vividly remember the day I decided to go on my first diet. I watched in the mirror with anticipation as I attempted to pull on a pair of my friend's jeans. I stopped two inches above my knees and in shock, looked down in hopes that I was the victim of a cruel optical illusion. At thirteen years old and maybe 112 pounds, I was stunned by my monstrous size, compared to my petite Asian friend. We had no understanding of the ethnic differences in body sizes. Looking back on that day, I shudder at the influence that one single image had on the next ten years of my life.

By age fourteen, I was already infected by the insidious need to be lean and perfect.

So my entire body renovation began. Dedicating every spare moment to counting calories and exercising, I missed out on many of the experiences that never return to a fourteen-year-old girl. My time spent with girlfriends became difficult. Although I would try to stay involved in the conversation, to enjoy the moment, to be the happy teenager I wanted to be, I couldn't get "outside of my own head." "Why did you let yourself eat that extra bagel at breakfast?" My thoughts would turn back to food and how I was going to redeem myself by burning off every last morsel that I had eaten. As my uneasiness grew, I'd make excuses to get away and be alone, just to alleviate my anxiety. I had control. I was thin. *I was lonely.* I got little joy out of being thin, yet letting go of control was not an option.

My days were rated good or bad based on what I ate, which, in turn, directly affected my moods. I was never outwardly mean or angry, but inside my head lived an evil dictator. I hid my feelings well behind a token smile, and although my family would sometimes comment on my preoccupation with weight, I was surprised that my friends said hardly a word. In hindsight, I now know that many other girls were going through similar struggles, so, together, we failed to notice one another's pain.

During my last year in high school I fell in love. Setting fear aside, I invited him into my home. I gave him the keys to both my heart and my body. "I have decorated perfectly," I thought. "*My* house is now *his* house." A comforting, warm belief until I learned the hard way that many eighteen-year-old males are quite happy in *any* house, with *any* decor, and with as *many* houses as physically possible. I was completely shattered and my self-esteem plummeted.

My inner voice raged, "You weren't good enough for him. What made you think that you were so special?" I let one person's immaturity and dishonesty confirm my self-judging beliefs and, soon after, my dieting days changed to more drastic measures. I began to force myself to vomit. I know that the word *vomit* paints a graphic picture, but to call it *purging* downplays my experience—especially when you look at the literal meaning of the word *purge*. To *purge* is to *become pure or clean, to rid oneself of guilt*. I was doing the opposite. At the time, I was a textbook eating-disorder case. White, upper-middle class upbringing, divorced parents, a list of relatives that suffered from alcoholism (there is a proven hereditary correlation between eating disorders and alcoholism), and, oh yes, not to leave out my people-pleasing personality. Add a broken heart to the equation and *wham!* By eighteen years of age I was living in a lonely, self-loathing, obsessive state of misery. Today's textbook case is no longer such a narrowly defined demographic. Eating disorders can affect any of us. They don't discriminate.

The irony behind my disorder was that I was seen as a young, healthy, smart fitness instructor—even respected for my pursuit of health at such a young age. I would berate myself: "You are a fraud. Why can't you just get yourself together?" This added more shame to the lie I was living. I was anxious that others might find out, lonely from keeping my disorder a secret, and ashamed of my sneaky and dishonest behavior—the two traits I despised most. I struggled for years with bulimia in isolation and frustration even though I knew I was destroying the beautiful house with which I had been blessed. Where was the foundation to this crumbling body and soul that I called home?

Several years later, while enjoying a weekend hiking trip, I found myself atop a rugged mountain peak, overlooking an astonishing view. Overly confident on the descent, I lost control, my feet moving me so quickly down the steep slope that my only salvation from the impending cliff was to sacrifice my body to the jagged rocks beneath me, in order to save myself from going over. Tumbling, punctured, and ripped open, I stopped falling. I had only one thought: "Thank God! I'm ALIVE," and the rest, I knew, were merely details.

It was in that bloody and bruised moment that I finally had a vivid yet peaceful glimpse of my foundation, *my spirit*. I was overwhelmed and humbled with joy and appreciation for all that surrounded me: the rugged mountains reaching for a cobalt-blue sky, my pounding heart echoing in my ears, the expression of relief washing over my brother's face as he packed snow into my wounds. For one unforgettable moment I was truly grateful for the value and beauty of my life, my body, my home.

Where Did My Healing Begin?

Healing does not happen overnight, nor does it happen, for that matter, in a ten-second, life-threatening fall down a mountainside. I had been making a slow emotional descent for years, creating a spiritual void that would take many unforgettable moments to fill back up. I demanded to feel whole again. I was no longer willing to live with the life-depriving emotions that had become my reality. I missed the parts of myself that brought me joy, but after so many lost years I didn't know where I was. What did I need to do to become whole again?

My first step was to take a hard, honest look at my beliefs. My judging thoughts had created a reality that I could no longer stand. For years, I had been unconsciously reinforcing these damaging beliefs, so I needed to accept that change would not happen immediately. It was going to take effort in order to achieve a state of *effortlessness*. I started learning, questioning, reading, and soul-searching. I studied psychology, kinesiology, sociology, and any other "ology" that helped me gain knowledge on my quest for wholeness. Drawing on many different disciplines, I used this information to create a powerful, foolproof recipe that empowered me to live my life *on purpose*. Although there were difficult moments confronting that inner dictator—a voice both loud and strong—as long as I turned to my personal recipe for inspiration, direction, and support, that oppressive voice eventually became inaudible. I didn't need to think of tomorrow or next week or next year, just the day's purpose. Although I wasn't always making *daily* progress, I refused to give up on myself. Whether it took ten months or ten years to feel whole again, I had faith that it was worth it—and it was. The rewards are priceless: a sense of freedom, the courage to forgive, non-judgmental love, and peace of mind.

My issues with food and body size faded away when I began to see perfection in all of my imperfections—eating disorder, waist size, and all! This isn't exactly the message fed to us by our society. Instead of starting a new and improved diet, my only job was to reinforce self-acceptance through actions that supported this belief—actions that defined *who I really was*. Like many of you, I, too, had originally started a diet wanting to lose weight. In the process, however, what I lost was the spirit of who I am. *This was the real disorder.*

Anyone who has struggled with her weight knows the pain of desiring freedom—freedom from thinking about food, freedom to know peace and balance in both body and mind, and freedom to spend energy pursuing personally fulfilling lives. I progressed from an innocent dieter looking to drop a few pounds, to becoming a young woman with an eating disorder. My quest had left me dangerously lost for years. Not surprisingly, most women who suffer from eating disorders first began by adhering to a restrictive diet.

As I stand here now with so many wonderful and painful memories living in this "house," I feel a deep respect for the gift that I have been given—my body. How I take care of it is my gift to the Giver. *This is why I choose health*. I try to eat foods that feed my cells with life, to go running especially if it is raining, and to laugh at myself for being so damn human. I still have challenging days, as we all do, but I have learned one hard-earned truth that I challenge you to act upon: Honor the quiet part of yourself that urges you to learn, grow, seek, and love. Your body and mind will follow suit and you'll rediscover your foundation, your *spirit*.

As you learn to cement your foundation daily with gratitude for all that you are, committing to a healthier lifestyle becomes a natural way to honor and nurture your whole self in body, mind, and spirit. Use this book as your guide and learn how to appreciate your physical body, feed your mind with empowering thoughts, and give your spirit the invaluable strength to withstand the storm.

CHAPTER TWO

Accepting the Challenge

Are You a Member of *The Diet Club*?

I WAS ONCE A most favored, loyal, and tormented member of *The Diet Club*, and with only a hint of apology, I believe that if you are reading this book, then you, too, may be a silent member. Welcome to the club—and guess what? No initiation fees!

Most new members become part of the club for free by passively adopting the messages of our diet-focused-body-conscious-media-crazed society. The power these messages have on how we *think* our bodies should look are insidious and complex, and woven into the very fabric of our culture. We sign the contract without consciously examining the mentality behind this ingrained belief. A concise oversimplification of the message would read something like this:

First, you must have the body. Slim. Lean. Strong. Sexy. Then you are permitted to reap society's rewards—respect, a successful career, a loving man who desires you, and personal validation as a strong-willed, competent, bathing-suit-wearing, free-spirited female!

It may seem like a fruitful endeavor, innocent at first: Just drop ten, twenty-five, sixty pounds—pick any number that suits you—and soon enough you will be in the game once again, proving your worth both as a woman and a human being. Club members know that weight loss is the only key to happiness. Unfortunately, many innocent dieters are led astray by first adopting this twisted belief. Ultimately, remaining a member of the Diet Club proves to be extremely costly, for membership dues can last a lifetime, constantly withdrawing inspiration and joy from the otherwise-rich bank account of our souls.

The contract that we sign in order to become a Diet Club member fails to provide us with the horrific statistics of what is really happening in the minds and hearts of many of us caught in a body-beautiful world.

- **61 percent** of adult Americans, both male and female, are overweight. About **one third (34 percent)** are obese, meaning that they are 20 percent or more above normal, healthy weight. Many of these people have binge eating disorder.

- It is *conservatively* estimated that **ten million** people suffer from eating disorders in the United States and Canada alone.

- Anorexia and bulimia primarily affect people in their teens and twenties, but clinicians report both disorders in children **as young as 6** and individuals **as old as 76**.

- **90 percent** of those struggling with eating disorders are female.

- Binge eating disorder seems to occur almost equally in males and females, although males are not as likely to feel guilty or anxious after a binge as women.

- **15 out of every 100** young women have some kind of disordered eating patterns.

- **Six million** young people are sufficiently overweight to endanger their health. Another five million children are borderline, and the problem grows larger every year.[1]

- There are **300,000** deaths a year attributed to obesity.[2]

---

[1]For extensive information regarding children and obesity, see www.obesity.org.

[2]The American Obesity Association backs this statistic, although there has been a lot of controversy over this particular number. For more detailed information click "editorial" on www.obesity.org.

All other statistics are quoted from ANRED, Anorexia Nervosa and Related Eating Disorders. ANRED is affiliated with NEDA, National Eating Disorders Association. See the Resources section on page 172 for more information.

Note: Determining accurate statistics is difficult because most people with these problems tend to be secretive, denying that they even have a disorder. I am one example that has gone unrecorded in the statistics (until the printing of this book, I suppose). Additionally, physicians are not required to report eating disorders to health agencies, so even if I had discussed my disorder with my doctor, I still could have slipped through the statistical cracks. Unfortunately, there is no way of knowing exactly how many people are actually affected.

The Role of Fashion Magazines and the Media

Whether we want to admit it or not, the media has an enormous effect on our beliefs. The fashion and beauty industries are not just selling us products; they are selling us entire images of how a woman should look and act. A recent psychological study found that 70 percent of women felt depressed, guilty, and shameful after looking at a fashion magazine for only three minutes. If this type of advertising is so detrimental to our self-esteem, why does it still dominate the media? One reason—*it works!*

How do you feel when you see a magazine full of ads featuring beautiful, thin models representing the *everywoman?* Ads depicting daughters, employees, wives, entrepreneurs, mothers, and college students selling us *stuff* so that we, too, may be as successful, beautiful, happy, stylish, sexy, smart, soft-skinned, white-toothed, etc., as they? Do you actually believe that the women you see portrayed in the media epitomize the women you see, talk to, and live with everyday? Of course not, we're not *that* gullible. We recognize that these carefully selected females are chosen in order to sell a product, an idea, an image. However, advertisers aren't naive either. Extensive research goes into targeting a particular market: you and me. Although we may consciously know that very few women have "model" looks, many of us still *subconsciously* compare ourselves to the women in fashion and beauty magazines, or worse, to the women in the new genre of men's magazines, such as *Maxim, Stuff, FHM,* and others.

The more we submerge ourselves in the fabricated beliefs of the advertising world, the more likely we are to drown in our own self-judgment and self-pity. Our good intentions to improve health and lose weight are heavily overshadowed by the incredible pressure to be more attractive, *now,* dictated to us by the unrealistic standards of a media-infused society. As a result, our emotional and spiritual well-being suffers greatly.

When reading magazines or watching TV commercials, try to be conscious of how these fabricated female ideals make you feel. Just being aware of how these insidious messages affect our thoughts gives us the power to stop these seemingly transparent messages from slipping into our subconscious beliefs.

Mandatory Club Policy:
All members must discriminate against personal
imperfection!

Answer the following questions as truthfully as possible to find out if you are a current Diet Club member. Pause long enough to personalize or expand on the feelings created by each one. In this exercise, it's not important whether you are five pounds or 150 pounds over your ideal weight because the beliefs that you hold about your body carry far more weight than any number you may see on the scale:

- Do you often look in the mirror and cringe at the appearance of your thighs (stomach, breasts, butt . . .)?

- When you encounter more fit or lean individuals do you feel inferior or envious?

- If there were less of you, would you be loved more?

- Do you avoid certain social situations that may draw attention to your body?

- Do you avoid social engagements where you will be tempted with food choices that you may be unable to avoid?

- Do you associate guilt or shame with eating certain foods?

- Are your intimate sexual moments negatively affected by how you feel about your body?

- Do you associate your level of happiness with your weight? (Even if you are only five or ten pounds heavier than you'd like to be?)

- Are your judgments of "good" and "bad" days dependent on food choices?

- Do you believe that by losing weight your life will become perfect?

- Do you think that your weight stops you from achieving your dreams and goals?

- Do you feel that you will never be satisfied with your body?

"Yes" answers are the sign of a true member. "Yes" answers reflect the damaging, judging, and unloving beliefs that we hold about ourselves. Analyze the questions to which you answered "yes." What are you reinforcing? Do you realize that you are discriminating against yourself? This type of harsh self-judgment leaches joy from our lives in every way imaginable. Would you instill these negative emotions onto a loved one, an innocent child, or even a stranger? Of course not. Yet we viciously and relentlessly injure the quiet, beautiful aspects of who we are.

Positive information may be trying to reach us, but are we blocking it? If we incessantly judge our bodies, our lives, and ourselves, then it becomes increasingly difficult to wholeheartedly accept even the most genuine compliment. Our minds are the final judge—the gates guarding our experience of life. What thoughts do your gates allow in? What joyous things are they turning away? What beliefs are perpetuating your current reality?

In order to cancel our membership to the Diet Club and end the struggle with weight, we must first become aware of the power of our thoughts. The body-beautiful mentality reflected in the media is not likely to change anytime soon, but we *can* take responsibility for how we internalize the images that are constantly being shoved at us. As we become better gatekeepers, we start to challenge the beliefs that have kept us from experiencing long-term weight loss and emotional freedom.

Gathering the Ingredients!

I am offering you my recipe—what has worked for me—from which you will adopt your own personal formula. You may feel skeptical at this point. Have faith, it will pay off. No matter how seemingly small, anything that expands our awareness has inherent value. I was, and still am, voracious about learning: reading, listening, and studying anyone who has something to say about healthy living, self-growth, spirituality, or psychology. I don't have to agree with all of the information, but instead, I extract what is helpful for me—*what speaks to me*. Therefore, extract the parts of this book that are useful to you, whether it be a single quote or all eleven chapters, and make it part of your own voice.

In addition to the important information in this book, there are three interactive chapters that request your participation. If you want to create change in your life, these exercises should not be skipped. Although these questions may take some time to complete, the more detailed information that you can draw from yourself, the more bountiful your recipe will be. Take your time. You do not have to complete these questions in one sitting. Enjoy.

CHAPTER THREE

Challenging Your Beliefs—
Renata's Story

*One person with a belief is equal to a
force of ninety-nine with only interests.*

—John Stuart Mill

WHEN RENATA WAS finally referred to me through her doctor, she was exhausted and discouraged. It was her third experience with a personal trainer, and although she had physically shown up for the appointment, I could see in her eyes that she still hadn't quite arrived. Who could blame her for her lack of enthusiasm? Two years prior, Renata had decided to lay down her hard-earned money on "personal trainer number one." A library of diet plans had already failed her. Just looking at those cardboard-boxed, pre-packed meals made her stomach rumble for anything fried, flaky, or Alfredoed. She had lost count of the number of times that she had fallen off the fitness bandwagon. Spiritually hungry and emotionally bruised, Renata was convinced that she was a lazy,

unmotivated person who would simply have to pay someone to FORCE her to eat well and exercise.

Renata's first trainer accepted her theory about why she
needed assistance. PT #1 did everything right, technically.
There was a basic fitness evaluation, followed by some diet
suggestions. Written fitness goals were sealed with appointment bookings—three times per week for the next three
months—and Renata wrote a check for $1,800. Renata
showed up. She exercised. She attempted to *be good* with
her eating. She even experienced moments of inspiration,
just like she had felt when she was good on the first few
days of a new diet.

However, as time went on, she often found herself re-
scheduling appointments or showing up late. When asked
about her diet progress, she felt guilty for not doing better,
and, although PT #1 was supportive, Renata began to feel
dependent on her trainer for her success. The *pay to be
forced to exercise* plan was not helping her during the other
twenty-three hours of the day when her trainer was not with
her. Maybe she needed five days a week? It was worth the
money, wasn't it? It was for health, right? Yet Renata's
growing dread prior to her appointments was far too rem-
iniscent of forced attendance in ninth-grade gym class.
Renata knew that something was still missing in her
weight-loss equation. She just didn't know what "it" was.

Leaving her trainer for another, PT #2, Renata continued on her search for the magic cure. She experienced the
same initial enthusiasm followed by an even lower drop in
motivation. Although PT #2 was not wrong in his exercise

prescription, he was not able to address Renata's inability to follow through on the goals that, together, they had set. They discontinued their sessions, as PT #2 suggested that Renata wait until she was *really* ready to lose weight. Ashamed at her lack of progress, not to mention loss of money, she agreed. The appointment was over.

She now felt as if she had failed every possible weight-loss and fitness plan ever known to woman. Personal trainer #2's words whirled in her head. "Wait until I was *really* ready to lose weight?" To Renata, her readiness was obnoxiously evident in the twenty-two years of life she had spent constantly consumed by food, dieting, and the size of her body! She questioned the hypocrisy of how she could truly want to free herself from excess weight, yet choose to live in a manner that would not support this desire. Was she going to have to pay someone for the rest of her life in order to stay healthy? What would be next? More diets? Liposuction? Stomach stapling? She seriously doubted whether she would ever experience balance, peace of mind, or the joy of living in a healthy, fit body.

Now at age forty-two, Renata was feeling a deep sense of failure and desperation. She approached her doctor requesting a prescription for antidepressants. After conducting tests, Renata's doctor believed that in her case, prescription drugs would not solve Renata's issue with weight. Instead she requested that Renata speak to one more trainer. The physician knew of another trainer who had a different approach to losing weight. Thankfully, Renata agreed, so we met simply to talk.

Thirty minutes into the session, without even changing into her exercise attire, Renata began to have the most meaningful workout of her life. We began to challenge her beliefs on weight loss and her motivation to experience optimal health.

- Why did Renata even want to lose weight?

- Were her beliefs regarding weight loss really hers or simply accepted, ingrained, and reinforced years ago?

- Are overweight people less lovable?

- How did she think losing weight would make her feel?

- Did she ever experience these emotions in her life now?

- What does health and happiness *feel* like?

- How could she create these feelings more often in her life today, prior to losing weight?

- Why did she quit her routine when she began to make progress?

- What was she willing to do in order to reach her goal?

- What was she unwilling to do?

- What messages did the media force-feed her?

- What did she want to do with these messages?

Question after question we both began to get excited as we peeled away the layers of Renata's unexamined notions and beliefs about weight loss and body image. By questioning Renata's attitudes toward weight loss, it was evident that her belief system had been keeping her from experiencing the very things that she truly wanted for herself. Regardless of her weight, how did she want to feel about her life? As she identified the emotions that she wanted to experience, she began to recognize how lost she had become. It was as if she was suffering an identity crisis. She had been acting in a manner that did not support her higher beliefs about who she really was. Her inability to lose weight was not the source of Renata's unhappiness. Instead, her desperation came from the spiritual void produced from the twenty-two years she'd spent measuring her own worth based upon the size of her waist. She had empowered the scale to determine how she was doing as a human being, yet *the spirit of who you are is unweighable*.

Renata's story strikes a chord for many Diet Club members. By allowing the scale gods to determine our level of happiness, this powerless belief becomes the source of our dissatisfaction, not the excess pounds. In fact, losing weight under this presumption can be very disappointing. If a smaller body is your main drive to becoming happy, you may in fact reach your goal only to ask, "Is that it? Shouldn't I now be feeling a sense of fulfillment in my life? Why has nothing really changed?" Regaining lost weight becomes inevitable.

Although the physical experience of a lighter, fit body is wonderful, it is not the true *source* of joy. Experiencing joy is available to us the moment we wake up. Joy is an attitude. It is a conscious choice. Think about it. It's 8:00 A.M. and you just woke up. That's the first good thing to be joyous about. You are safe, warm, and have an infinite selection of foods to choose from for breakfast. What is not to be grateful for? Oops, bad question. Why? Because if we look for an answer there is always something negative on which to focus our attention. Again, we have a choice.

How Do You Choose to Focus Your Energy?

There is not a day that goes by (for any of us) without potential frustrations, irritations, or disappointments. Whether it is the number we see stepping onto the scale, the number in our bank account, or larger issues like feeding the hungry, world peace, and environmental conservation, there will always be things to complain about. But *how* we focus our attention determines how we feel, and how we feel—our state of mind—powerfully influences our actions and attitudes.

How does this scenario make you feel: You planned to meet your friend at a restaurant, yet she is over twenty minutes late. As you are waiting for her to show up, what thoughts enter your mind? "Maybe she doesn't care enough to be on time. Perhaps she was in a car accident. She's probably shopping for a gift for me—how great!" Think about how each of these potential explanations makes you feel. Each perspective, regardless of whether it's the right one, creates a feeling that leads to a reaction. Some feelings are obviously more empowering than others.

What is your attitude toward living a healthy, fit life? What are your beliefs? If the internal focus is, "I will always be dissatisfied with my body," or "I am not strong enough to commit to long-term health," chances are you will continue to focus on the external feedback that makes these beliefs true. There will always be a reason why *now* is a bad time to exercise. There will always be someone more attractive, younger, and slimmer to threaten your self-esteem if you think that way, just as there are infinite excuses to condone overeating.

After driving to work in thick traffic for the past two years, Sandra starts thinking. "I hate this drive to work. I listen to the news and it is so terrible that I don't even feel safe in my own city anymore. Since it's dark when I get home, I can't go for a walk outside, even though I have been sitting for over eleven hours today. I deserve to watch some television and eat my favorite ice cream just to get away from thinking about tomorrow." These are legitimate frustrations with which we can all identify. A change in focus, however, takes Sandra on a whole new path. "My travel time is bothering me. I can get up earlier and exercise near work before I start my day and miss traffic entirely. I can listen to my favorite music or books on tape while driving, and start to walk during my lunch, perhaps with others who have similar frustrations." An exciting and creative part about being human is the infinite number of ways in which we are able to look at life. There is always another angle, view, or opinion from which to conceptualize our experience. Our reality is in our own hands.

When you think about losing weight, what are the first thoughts that come to mind? Is it "I don't know why I bother doing this. I always give up a few days into my plan anyway," or "Here we go again. I wonder if I'll even get to Friday before blowing it?" How does this make you feel? Pessimistic? Overwhelmed? Defeated? Isn't it far more motivating and exciting to focus on the favorable feelings? "At first it may be tough to implement healthy changes in my lifestyle, but soon enough I'm going to feel fantastic!" We control the focus of our thoughts. Our reality is shaped not by what life presents us but rather by how we choose to view it. Therefore, taking control of how we view our bodies, our health, and our *selves* gives us the freedom to choose our experience of life.

There are unlimited things in life to focus on, and, as most of us know all too well, there is a limited amount of time in any given day. Given this fact, how do you choose to view your life's circumstances? On what do you focus your time? What do you often think about?

More specific to weight loss and health, how do you choose to feel about yourself? As you watch the Sunday running club pass by your doorstep, do you feel discouraged or inspired? Do you spend time dwelling on why you are not small-boned and 5'11" or do you focus on your own beautiful body, mind, and spirit? Are you grateful for your health, your miraculous body, and the wonderful life that you have been given? Which focus motivates and inspires healthy living? You have the choice.

Shifting Focus to See the *Whole* Picture

Experiencing peace of mind, joy, fulfillment, and deep contentment in one's life is *not* synonymous with having a twenty-four-inch waist. In order to receive these gifts, we must stop bowing to the scale gods and, instead, create a life focused on the actions and behaviors that reflect our deepest desires. How do you start to create a new path toward a more inspired life? First, take a closer look at yourself and ask: How do I want my life to unfold? With whom do I want to share my life—family, a partner, children, friends, pets? What do I love to do in my leisure time? What do I get excited about? What makes me laugh? What qualities do I admire in a person? What do I admire about myself? When I am old, how do I want to remember my life? What makes me feel alive?

When we make the choice to create a life that excites, nurtures, and soothes our souls, then procrastination, overeating, and inactivity can no longer Band-Aid our aching hearts. Yet beyond creating a life that expresses *all that you are,* you have the power to change your attitude in an instant. It's called an *attitude of gratitude*. It's so simple, and yet so underused. If we can look at our lives this very moment and be grateful for the abundance, freedom, wealth, and beauty that is *already* in our lives, then our motivation to lose weight shifts. We feel empowered instead of inferior. We are inspired rather than threatened. We see abundance in our life, not lack of it. We want to do *loving* things for our bodies, instead of punishing them with inactivity, restrictive diets, judging thoughts, or junk food. We no longer feel that we *have* to lose weight in order to feel happy, attractive, or successful, but instead, we are empowered to take care of our bodies, minds, and souls—in whatever form that may be.

Struggling with weight year after year, feeling deprived and frustrated, is not experiencing our true essence. Yet when we live with a sense of gratitude, and take responsibility for how our lives play out, then we reap the wonderful rewards of purposeful living. We have faith and trust in ourselves, we feel inspired and energetic, we have a sense of inner peace, and we have direction in our lives. We are more patient and forgiving, and we choose to treat our bodies with respect. Aren't these some of the key motivational ingredients to the long-term success of a health and fitness program? Here are some examples of how motivation changes when perspective shifts:

MOVING FROM:
I need to lose weight to be fulfilled and happy.
TO:
I am losing weight because I am happy and grateful for my life, today.

MOVING FROM:
I want to look a certain way on the outside to make me feel better on the inside.

TO:
My body is a physical expression of how I feel inside—
free, healthy, active, light, and empowered.

This shift in awareness makes all the difference in how we
fulfill our desires. We are creating flow *into* our lives. We
are finally tapping into our true essence.

Remembering "Who You Are" Is the Most Important Weight-Loss Exercise You Will Do

Reconnecting with the things that are important to you
in your life and identifying what brings you joy, peace,
excitement, and love is the first step to getting back to your
true essence. Think about how great it feels to be inspired—
naturally aligned with your purpose and focusing positive
energy toward your well-being. When your daily reality
reflects your inner truth, there is no struggle to stay motivated. You are in sync with yourself, free to experience the
effortlessness of intrinsic motivation—*the source of motivation that is inherent in every one of us*.

Like many of us, Renata had continually skipped this
crucial first step of looking inward, focusing solely on the
physical, external factors regarding weight loss. Calories in,
calories out. The right diet. The frequency and intensity of
exercise. The attempt at every new fitness or diet trend in
the hopes of finding tricks to keep her willpower strong.
Yet time and again she always dropped out. Why? Because

she was giving herself away. Diets became punishing. Exercise became a chore. Feelings of failure overpowered her goals and, ultimately, trying to lose weight became a great source of pain. She felt she was losing herself.

I did not give Renata a magic cure. She did not wake up the next day and pull on a pair of jeans from her high-school days. Instead, she left with something real. One stride in the right direction, Renata took responsibility for how her life had been unfolding and committed to *herself,* to get back to her true essence.

Throughout our following sessions, we continued to work on both the mental and physical habits that, for the last twenty-two years, had left Renata feeling totally disconnected from her body. I merely asked the questions; it was Renata who searched for the right information. Together we combined these ingredients to create a daily recipe for her success. As Renata began to connect with this internal source of inspiration, she was no longer waiting for the scale to dictate when it was okay to feel good. Feeling gratitude for her life, Renata approached each day with a sense of accountability toward herself and her life. Her only daily job was to remain committed to nurturing herself in body, mind, and spirit. By following her own individual plan, Renata remained intrinsically motivated to honor her weight-loss goals. Soon, the issues that blocked her from staying motivated became impotent. For the first time, Renata's weight loss became both an external and internal expression of who she was. The struggle was gone and Renata was back.

The weight struggle is very real when we praise the scale as our personal deity, yet scales merely measure objects, not human worth. Scales cannot measure excitement, freedom, or the beauty of smiling eyes. We are in control of our happiness. The scale cannot weigh our spirit, it is immeasurable. When we find this connection within, the struggle will cease.

CHAPTER FOUR

Getting Back to You

*How do we get reconnected with our true essence, stay
motivated, and end the struggle with food and weight?*

Exercise #1
Writing Your Story

I SHARED MY STORY at the beginning of this book
for one reason. It was incredibly useful for *me*. I had
originally written most of my experience in a journal years
ago, and in doing so, it helped me to take responsibility for
how my life had progressed, mistakes and all. The purpose
of looking at our past is not to judge it, deny it, or seal the
fate of our future—but instead, to simply change our perception of it in order to move forward. By objectively looking at what I had written, I was able to forgive myself for
the emotional and physical damage that I had put myself
through. Quite simply, I had been looking for life's beau-

tiful gifts, yet I didn't know how to find them. Understand-ably, I got lost. Today I have clear guidelines to direct me—spiritually, mentally, emotionally, and physically. By the time you reach the end of this book, you will have the tools to help yourself.

I encourage you to take some time to write your own story. Feel free to use any format with which you feel com-fortable. This exercise is for your eyes only, so try to be as thorough, honest, and reflective as you can. If you have a hard time getting started or get stuck along the way, use some of these questions to guide your writing:

- When did you first begin to have issues with food?
- When did you first start to gain excess weight?
- What was going on in your life?
- How did you feel about yourself?
- Are there any patterns in your story?
- What weight-loss methods have you tried?
- How did these different techniques make you feel?
- What have you learned?
- Where are you today?

Feel free to use the space provided in the Exercise section of the Appendix on pages 144–146. If you think you may need extra space or would like more privacy, use a journal or notebook. Personally, I like to use a separate notebook for two reasons: One, when I first start to brainstorm, my handwriting is so messy that I usually need a second draft for legibility, and two, my answers can remain private should I choose to pass the book on to a friend or client. Do whatever works for you.

Final comments on writing your story

Now that you have finished, you may feel somewhat emotional. Writing about the past inevitably brings up many memories, both painful and pleasurable ones. Try to refrain from judging what you have written. Just for today, leave it on the paper and let it go. Close this book for now. Tomorrow, with fresh eyes, reread your story along with the remainder of this chapter.

Leaving the Past Where It Belongs

As you begin to reflect on your story, you may find it helpful to apply the following insights. In fact, *what* you wrote is far less important than how you choose to look at it. If you took the time to write your story, yet continue to punish yourself for your history, then all you are doing is reliving past experiences. Failing to forgive ourselves is the fastest way to get into a rut. We gain the power to change ingrained patterns as soon as we recognize the futility of dwelling on the past. The information on the following pages can help you change your perception of past mistakes, propelling you into a new future.

Mistakes

· **We have made mistakes in the past, we will continue to make more of them in the future, and it's okay.**

Relationships, financial investments, diet plans, you name it—we don't *really* know how *anything* is going to work out. We constantly make choices in life without access to future information—it's called *living*. We are bound to make mistakes. Since we can't live without them, so to speak, we must learn to live with them. Accepting this fact frees us from the anguish and guilt of thinking, "If I had only done it *that* way instead. . . ." We did the best we could with the information that we had.

· **We grow, we love, and we heal in life when we are *experiencing* it.**

Our past is made up of millions of interactions—a constantly evolving collection of moments that has shaped our experience of life. Who said we were supposed to get it exactly right? What is *right* anyway? A life with no mistakes? No challenges? Life is spontaneous and uncertain— the very things that make it interesting. Why would we want it any other way? Making mistakes just proves that we are *in the game*. Good for us! Mistakes hurt, but the lessons are so precious. Since we can't experience life by passively watching it, we must be gentle with ourselves for not always scoring the game-winning goal, or for that matter, letting the "game-winner" get by us. Celebrate your humanness for taking the risk that led to making the mistake in the first place.

· **Failing to lose weight is not a mistake.**

What was your crime? Not being able to stick to a short-term, restrictive, unpractical food plan? You may not have had the right nutrition and health information. Perhaps you have never challenged your beliefs or tapped into what motivates you from the inside out. Unfortunately, there are horrific mistakes that happen in the world—failing to lose weight is *not* one of them. Keep things in perspective. Remember that the scale does not determine your worth!

· **What patterns emerge throughout your story?**

The measure of success is not whether you have a tough problem to deal with, but whether it's the same problem you had last year.

—*John Foster Dulles*

Pay attention to the problems and challenges that continue to plague your weight-loss efforts. The things that we are reluctant to address or change often contain the most valuable lessons. Ask yourself: What is really bothering me about this situation? Is there something that I need to learn?

What small thing can I do to break out of this pattern? If there is one thing that we always have, it is choice.

Elisabeth Kübler-Ross said, "Learn to get in touch with the silence within yourself, and know that everything in life has purpose. There are no mistakes, no coincidences; all events are blessings given to us to learn from."

Forgiveness

· **What do you need to forgive?**

What have you been doing to yourself that you need to forgive? Have you been supporting self-punishing thoughts? Feeding your body with junk food? Binge eating? Crash dieting? It may help to make a list.

· **Forgiving yourself is not the same as condoning the behavior.**

Just because you forgive yourself for attempting five crash diets in the last two years doesn't mean that you should repeat the same scenario this year. From years of personal judgment right up to last night's binge, forgive yourself, not the behavior.

· **Who is being hurt by your non-forgiveness?**

When we *choose* to not forgive ourselves for the past, *we* are the ones who suffer with frustration, guilt, and anger. In addition to self-inflicted pain, our loved ones also hurt for us. As my eating disorder progressed, I was not the only one suffering. My family suffered greatly, too. Yet as long as I continued to punish myself with judgment and guilt, they were powerless to help me. Forgiveness is the first step to healing. No one else can do it for you. If you have a hard time forgiving yourself, then, at first, do it for the ones who love you.

· **Create a clean slate in order to move forward.**

Get rid of the things that bring you pain. I found it liberating to stop buying a particular magazine that promoted ultra-thin models and fasting-type diets. I got rid of clothes that were either too large or too small for my body. I became aware of certain coworkers who brought out my self-deprecating thoughts. Be mindful of the things, situations, or people that challenge your own self-forgiveness.

· **Failing to forgive perpetuates failure.**

When it comes to healing our food and body issues, forgiveness is not something we can save for later when we *reach* our goals. It doesn't work that way. I didn't forgive myself *after* I got better; I forgave myself while I was *still* sick. Out of shame or denial, we may not feel worthy of forgiveness. Again, just because we forgive ourselves doesn't mean that we accept our current conditions—we are all free to change. But by accepting ourselves without judgment, we actually begin to move forward. We are no longer condemned to stay stuck where we are. Again: *forgive yourself, not the behavior.*

Facing Fear

Courage is resistance to fear, mastery of fear—not absence of fear.

—Mark Twain

A great acronym many people have used to describe FEAR is **F**alse **E**vidence **A**ppearing **R**eal. Fears are stumbling blocks to rediscovering who we are. They show up at unexpected times for unusual reasons. The fear of failing is the greatest fear keeping us from being truly spectacular. Could it be that we associate failing with the most painful emotion—being unloved? Our fears are the ultimate blinders that keep us from seeing our own beautiful truth and experiencing all that we desire. For example, Dorothy, in the *Wizard of Oz,* faced her fear, pulled back the dark curtain using the strength of her faith, and found that nothing was there. When we choose to look behind our own curtain of fears, once exposed, they become less ominous. Marianne Williamson says it so beautifully in the following quote from her 1992 book, *Return to Love.* Nelson Mandela later included this passage as part of his 1994 inaugural speech.

Our deepest fear is not that we are inadequate.

Our deepest fear is that we are powerful beyond measure.

It is our light, not our darkness, that most frightens us.

We ask ourselves, who are we to be gorgeous, talented, and fabulous?

Actually, who are you not to be? You are a child of God!

Your playing small doesn't serve the world.

There is nothing enlightened about shrinking so that people don't feel insecure around you. We were born to manifest the glory of God that is within us.

It's not just in some of us; it's in everyone. And as we let our light shine, we unconsciously give other people permission to do the same.

As we are liberated from our own fear, our presence automatically liberates others.

Reread this passage when you feel as though your current thought patterns are beginning to shadow over your own incredible light.

Moving Forward Fearlessly

Leaving the past behind enables us to act in the present. The present is the only place we *can* start. Right this moment we can make a difference. This is why it is so important for us to write our stories and begin to recognize some of the beliefs that have landed us where we are today. If we continue along the same path, nothing will change. As Einstein said, "Insanity is doing the same thing over and over, and expecting a different result." When it comes to weight loss, many of us can relate to Albert's description of madness.

This next exercise focuses on whether losing weight is actually worth your energy. It does not determine if you *should* lose weight, or try to convince you why you would benefit from doing so. I certainly can't guarantee you that losing weight will live up to your expectations. It may, but it very well may not. The only person who knows whether you really want to change your current behavior is you. These three sets of questions will help you decide if the effort to lose weight is a venture worth choosing.

There are no rules for how you approach these questions. If you feel like only answering some of them, fine. It may be that some don't apply to you. They are only intended to bring clarity to your thoughts and beliefs surrounding weight loss. Read each question through and then answer those that grab your attention. If you have answered similar questions before, remain open-minded to the possibility that you could have a different response now. We are often conditioned to give a particular answer whether or not it actually reflects our true beliefs. As long as you are honest about how you *really* feel, this exercise will be of value to you.

Exercise #2

QUESTION ONE: Why do you want to lose weight?

Why is it important to you—or is it? Are you concerned about your health? Are you trying to make others happy? Do you want to look better in a bathing suit? What is your primary motivation? What do you think will happen in your life when you lose weight? Other than the size of your body, what will change? Whether you consider them silly or serious, list all of the reasons why you want to lose weight or improve your overall health and well-being. (See the Exercise section of the Appendix on page 147.)

QUESTION TWO: Are you willing to challenge yourself and work at your goal?

Making the commitment to improve our health takes effort. Change, for many of us, can bring up emotions that we may not feel comfortable experiencing. Are the reasons why you want to change important enough to you that you are willing to work at reaching your goal? Whether you are changing your physical lifestyle (activity level or eating habits) or altering ingrained beliefs about weight loss, are you willing, at times, to feel challenged? Are you willing to be courageous and have faith when walking this new path in order to experience your true essence?

QUESTION THREE: Are you willing to accept, love, and nurture your whole self—independent of weight loss?

This is a tough one. Most of us don't want to accept ourselves, let alone love ourselves, when we don't like the way we look. Yet before we can lose weight permanently we *must* celebrate our whole self—beyond our thighs. What actually makes a person lovable? Is it just his or her body? Beyond the physical, what is attractive about you? What do family, friends, and coworkers like about you? Do you think your attitude toward your own body is loving? Are you willing to change the way you see yourself?

When we challenge the beliefs we hold about the size of our bodies, we become conscious of the impact these thoughts have had on our entire life. These answers are powerful clues to help us determine the source of our motivation. Right or wrong, they have led us to where we now stand. From this day forward, we get to determine how our lives unfold.

Don't be frustrated if there are contradictions in your answers. Our beliefs are often filled with mixed messages. We are complex creatures; being ambiguous is part of what makes humans so interesting. Just be aware that, at times, you may have been acting from beliefs that conflict with one another. Take a good look at your answers. Ask from your heart, "Which beliefs have nurtured me? Which ones have harmed me?" Your heart knows the right answer. As we begin to identify the beliefs that have fed our insecurities, we start to expose and discard our damaging fears. Keep the beliefs that have served you well. They will continue to motivate growth. In every moment, every day, we are acting out our life's choices, based on both helpful and disabling beliefs. *It is essential to distinguish between the two in order to establish a more fruitful path.*

To Lose or Not to Lose . . .

What if, while answering these questions, you realize that the desire to lose weight was never yours in the first place? Congratulations! By looking at your answers, you may see through your prior motivations and for *empowering* reasons, no longer have the desire to lose weight for others. Wonderful! Invest the time and energy pursuing other goals. This is your life and you have the choice. However, if you determine, based on your own personal reasons, that losing weight and improving your health is a genuine desire of yours, do not deny yourself this truth. When we are faced with challenges, it's very easy to trick ourselves into believing that what we want is not attainable or valuable. Behind the denial of our desires there is usually a fear lurking about. As you begin to seek out potential fears, remember there are endless types—fear of failure, fear of change, fear of success, fear of getting more attention, and so on. What fears do you need to face in order to move forward?

Working toward a healthier lifestyle requires effort— not only in changing our eating habits and daily activity levels, but in our thinking patterns, too. Ultimately, suppressing our desires becomes a far more difficult task than actually committing to healthier living. Creating a lifestyle that promotes weight loss is actually a lot easier than many people believe, but before you begin the physical part of your journey toward greater health and well-being, you must first dismantle the biggest obstacle to weight loss success—the *ego threat*.

CHAPTER FIVE

The Ego Threat—
Our Greatest Obstacle

IT'S ESTIMATED THAT 90 percent of women are dissatisfied with some aspect of their body, 70 percent are preoccupied with their weight, and 40 percent of women are yo-yo dieting. These statistics show that if our goal is to make peace with our bodies, we are failing miserably. Yet if we consider the growing number of women who are actually informed about nutrition and exercise, it's clear that we can't attribute our lack of success to insufficient knowledge.

Armed with accurate information and a genuine desire to improve ourselves, how can we still be so vulnerable to fall prey to the trappings of self-doubt and discouragement? We often start weight loss and exercise programs "on fire," motivated and inspired, but at the first sign of temptation, we break down and deviate from our health plan. How can we avoid giving in to immediate gratification? What threatens our good intentions?

A *threat* is an expression of intent to inflict pain, injury, or punishment. Many advertising companies sell products by using threats as a form of marketing. Picture the dandruff commercial that depicts a woman turning away from her dark-haired date stating that "He'd be great . . . if it weren't for those flakes!" Threat: buy this shampoo or be alone and single forever. Not exactly life-threatening, but nonetheless a threat to squelch our social lives. This is a simple example, but what actually threatens our motivation to improve health and lose weight permanently?

The threats I am referring to are non-fatal in nature, yet nonetheless powerful in their effect on our mental, emotional, and spiritual well-being. More appropriately, I will refer to them as *ego* threats. Used in this sense, *ego* refers to the traits that give us a social identity—the ways in which we label one another and ourselves, based, for example, on our cultures, our ages, how we look, the shape of our bodies, how we think or want others to view us, our role with family, friends, and lovers, and our job titles, to name a few. These labels are vulnerable to change, and as our lives unfold, we constantly reevaluate and adjust our ego identities. We are constantly reshaping the *ego* part of ourselves, yet the true essence of who we are does not change.

So who are we, if we cannot be defined by our ego labels? Here is an exercise that was first introduced to me during a seminar with Deepak Chopra. It is aimed to help us recognize the *non-ego* part of our identities that never changes. Close your eyes and ask yourself the following questions. Give yourself time with each question, spending fifteen to twenty seconds with each. Just let feelings or images surface. "Who am I? What do I want? What is my purpose?" What adjectives pop into your thoughts? Continue repeating these three questions in your mind until you come up with a mind full of answers.

Now think back to when you were a child. Imagine yourself at age six or seven. Picture that girl in your mind. See yourself growing up over the years. Age ten, then thirteen . . . fifteen . . . eighteen, and continue. Ask yourself the same three questions, "Who am I? What do I want? What is my purpose?" Allow your memories to surface. Repeat these questions while reflecting on each stage of your life. What part of you has never changed? What answers are repeated? Can they be reduced to a single statement or word?

At our seminar, participants offered different adjectives and themes to describe their experiences, but when asked to reduce their list to one word, to one driving motivation, to one purpose, all 250 people sitting in that room agreed that it was *love*. At the core of "Who am I?" is love. "What have I always wanted?"—love. "What is my purpose?"— to love. Our lives are the unique expression of this purpose.

This exercise is just one simple way to look at our non-ego self, helping us to remember that our ego is the "clothing" we choose to wear over our true essence—the part of us that does not change. The clothing is a part of us, yet it is not *all that we are.*

All that said, understanding the ego's role and attempting to surpass its imaginary ability to grant worthiness is difficult. The social threat of being overweight in a culture obsessed with slim bodies is daunting, making our egos wince more often than we would like. It's easy to think of a few common ego threats:

· Exposing your naked body to a new love interest. Yes, without the covers.

· An upcoming beach vacation requiring a bathing-suit-clad body—leaving you only two weeks to morph into a new being.

· Being offered the seniors' menu when you are still ten years away from age sixty-five.

· An invitation to your high school reunion that cries out potential judgment of not only your body, but also of your marital status, career, and appearance.

You may feel that these scenarios are legitimate reasons to want to look good and lose weight, and they are! We are human, and not only do we need to be fulfilled spiritually and emotionally, but we want to look and feel great, too. But what if our ego becomes our only source of identity? What if we can't "separate the clothes from the woman"? When our realities become centered on this external shell, the true self is hidden. We are at the mercy of our ego threats.

When we sense that our egos are being attacked, feelings of jealousy, insecurity, and fear swell within us. Protecting ourselves from painful emotions becomes a full-time job. We work to keep our "ego clothing" from being torn or frayed and although these emotions surface in an attempt to shield pain, it is ineffective. We suffer anyway, trying to maintain our ego identities. Torn to shreds, we are unable to tap into our true essence. We lack inspiration. We lack motivation. Our actions do not represent our best intentions. Because we hurt, we soothe ourselves with food, with procrastination, or with apathy and self-pity. Ouch.

So the Pain Continues . . .

Indulging the ego with power gives it free rein to mask our true identity—our timeless self. Ego-driven, we turn to images and ideals outside of our heart, in order to find self-worth. In the media, for example, we are inundated daily with ego threats. Everywhere we look we see beautiful women with long legs, flowing hair, full breasts, little behinds, and tiny waists. Without the help of plastic surgery, the majority of these bodies wouldn't naturally exist, yet we are still deeply influenced by these images. It's shocking to think that among Hollywood actresses, a size four is now considered large! Will these trends undermine our satisfaction of living in a healthy size-eight, -ten, or -twelve body? What if size-four feet became fashionable? Would we think it's acceptable to shove our size-nine feet into size-four shoes? What if, God forbid, we should age? Would we feel desperate to look thirty years old at age sixty-five? My examples may *seem* extreme, but are they really? Look how far we have *already* been led.

If we allow external factors to determine our worthiness, self-acceptance can only be attained by surrendering to the ever-changing trends and ideals of the day. From this position, we constantly need to *prove* that we are attractive, successful, worthy, valuable, and lovable—instead of simply knowing it. This is not security or happiness—it's terrifying! So how can we step beyond our ego identities to be less vulnerable to the daily threats that undermine our inspiration and happiness? A small shift in consciousness is a fabulous start.

Conceptualizing Ourselves in a New Light

When we look at a newborn child, we see perfection. There is nothing a baby needs to prove, as she is already complete without any *ego clothing*. We, too, were once newborns, complete and perfect in every way. What makes us think that anything has changed? Of course we have grown up, developed our personalities, become knowledgeable, and have stored innumerable memories from our lives, yet we are still no less complete, no less perfect than the day we were born. But unfortunately, somewhere along the line, our ego made a judgment, and it's had an imperfect opinion of who we are ever since.

How would you feel right this moment if you knew that you were already considered perfect, just as you are? If you woke up each day and gave thanks for your *perfection*, how would this sense of gratitude affect your life?

Coming from this level of consciousness, what experiences would you want to have? In other words, if there was nothing for you to prove in life, nothing to fear, what would you want to experience?

Perhaps you'd decide that you would like the experience of living in a healthy and fit body. Would you want to be free from thinking obsessively about food and weight? You might also choose to have a life chock-full of nurturing, loving relationships, or maybe spend more of your free time pursuing personal passions. Maybe you would want enough money and time to travel. What else would you want to experience in your life? Give yourself a moment to think about it.

Now ask yourself, "Am I willing to do the work—spiritually, emotionally, and physically—to have this splendid 'wardrobe,' so that I can experience all the beautiful things that life has to offer?" Secondly, "Can I wear these clothes with gratitude and humility, relying on none of them to prove my completeness?"

Freedom comes when we can consistently answer "yes" to these two questions. Saying "yes" is a process, requiring an ongoing commitment to nurturing our *whole* selves.

When judgmental thoughts enter your mind, remember that you are a spiritual being invulnerable to the transient trends and opinions of the day. We can trust that, independent of societal pressures, our true essence çannot be altered. Being aware of our spiritual backbone allows us to take more risks and go after all of our desires. What kind of life do you want to live? The choice is yours. When we are in this state of awareness, ego threats become powerless, unable to shake our solid foundations.

CHAPTER SIX

The Ultimate Motivation

*If we all did the things we are capable of
doing, we would literally astound ourselves.*

—Thomas Edison

SAVE THIS CHAPTER for a time when you can relax, enjoy, and completely focus on yourself. Ready? Sink into your favorite chair and let's begin.

We all want to be endlessly and effortlessly motivated, acting with our *spiritual selves* in mind, in order to express the unlimited nature of our true essence: harmony, bliss, creativity, joy, truth, and natural perfection. Yet the energy required to stay motivated is often the most challenging factor. Remaining committed to self-improvement requires a level of discipline and motivation that is not always easy to attain, yet the effort taken to better ourselves most assuredly leads to satisfaction. Tapping into our *intrinsic* source of motivation is the most important factor in making this trip more successful.

Remember when, as a child, you were absorbed by your favorite game for hours? It was rewarding on its own, without the need for parental coercion. You were playing. It was effortless. Your own curiosity, excitement, and interest motivated you. You weren't focused on any particular reward; in fact, *participating* in the activity was in itself rewarding. You were intrinsically motivated to play.

As adults we still want to be intrinsically motivated. Instead of being motivated to *play,* however, we want the effortlessness and passion to spill over into *all* areas of our lives. It's easy to recognize people who are intrinsically motivated. They are those who are free from the influence of self-doubt, procrastination, or any other obstacle in the way of their happiness. In the face of adversity, they simply find a way to realize their goals. Imagine pursuing your dreams and passions with no need for external encouragement. Wouldn't our lives be so much more enjoyable and productive if we could rely solely on our own infinite sources of motivation to carry us through life, especially for those times when we just don't *feel* like working at it? Well, we can—it just takes a little searching.

What are some of the emotions that naturally motivate us? Regardless of the actual actions or behaviors that elicit these emotions, what do we all want to experience? Some of our intrinsic motivators are: *Freedom, excitement, joy, effortlessness, peace, gratitude, love, competence, creativity, serenity, elation, empowerment, bliss, inspiration, connectedness, happiness.* What others can you think of?

• • •

Now let's address the desire to lose weight. When we turn to personal trainers, exercise videos, diet support groups, fitness classes, and weight-loss books, what are we primarily looking for? Motivation! Many of these external motivators can, in fact, help us reach our goals, under one condition: we must be able to associate intrinsic rewards to the actions we take.

Here is a simple example: If a father pays his daughter, Judith, to get good grades in school, she is *extrinsically motivated* by money. If, during the process, she feels a sense of mastery and competence, she is likely to continue doing well in school after her father has stopped paying her. At that point, Judith has become intrinsically motivated to study and learn. Therefore, if changing a specific behavior doesn't come naturally at first, using external motivation to jump-start our own infinite source of motivation is the key. However, we usually quit or drop out when we are unable to find anything intrinsically motivating about a certain behavior, and, in time, external motivators become ineffective. Although losing weight is a much more complex issue than Judith and her grades, from a behavioral point of view, similar principles still apply. If you cannot find something enjoyable about exercising at your gym, at some point you'll stop going. If you feel deprived when eating a restrictive diet, one day you'll go off it. If each time you go running you experience pain, you'll eventually quit.

At times, we all need encouragement and support to

stay committed to our goals—the goals that will allow us to feel fit, light, healthy, and energetic. But as long as we believe that the key to staying motivated lies outside of ourselves, we will endlessly look for the fix—jumping into new diets, trends, and trainers to keep us "pumped up." It's as if we want someone else to direct us, someone else to plant the desire within us, someone else to expand our consciousness. Yet in order to achieve lifelong weight loss, we must be intrinsically motivated to stick to a healthier diet and exercise plan. Our weight loss success actually hinges on our *own* ability to elicit these positive emotions within ourselves. Although outside support can nurture our growth, it is ineffective as long as we neglect to first plant our own seeds. These next exercises will help you to pinpoint your personal intrinsic motivators.

As you begin the exercises in this section, try to approach your *self* in a spiritual light, as discussed in Chapter Five. Remember, there is nothing for you to prove in life, so how do *you* want it to be? What do you choose to experience? You are in control.

Exercise #3

QUESTION ONE: What does being fit and healthy feel like to you?

Recognizing the rewards and simple pleasures that healthy living brings to our life inspires us to act! We are tapping into our intrinsic motivators. In fact, if we can't even imagine the rewards of optimal well-being and weight loss, then a sedentary life, overeating, and giving in to immediate gratification will still be a comfortable choice.

Start by reflecting on the times in your life when you felt connected to your body—free to enjoy the pleasures of health and well-being—liberated from self-judgment. How did being healthy *feel*? What was it like to be in your body? How did your health affect your mental and emotional experience?

Imagine how your ideal self would feel living inside a healthy, fit body. In your mind, visualize how it feels to love and embrace the body in which you live. What are the rewards of honoring the self? How do you feel? What do you notice around you? How do you treat others? How do you treat yourself? What do you eat? How does your body feel as it moves?

Since this is an abstract question, I have included some of the inspiring feelings and satisfying moments that I experience when I am taking care of my physical health. Just reading this list reminds me of all the wonderful emotions and pleasures that come to me when I honor my health and fitness goals. To get started, you may choose to use some of these in your own "healthy list."

- loving the moment
- feeling strong
- taking action (however small)
- feeling light

- being inspired
- moving freely
- wanting everyone to succeed
- catching myself laughing from the depths of my belly
- savoring the fresh, sweet taste of fruit
- a sense of having time "on my side"
- waking from a restful sleep
- not worrying about the things I can't control
- enjoying small pleasures each day
- finding a positive way to look at things
- not getting upset in traffic
- noticing the beauty and perfection in everything
- being energized by the clean, salty ocean air
- walking in silence in the woods
- smelling the rain
- enjoying being touched
- getting "butterflies" when listening to a beautiful piece of music
- saying no to food that doesn't build health
- being relaxed
- experiencing a sense of quiet excitement
- going "with the flow"
- getting the giggles for no particular reason
- feeling confident
- being aware of thirst versus hunger
- feeling creative and curious
- standing tall
- noticing the "good" things in the mirror

- feeling a deep sense of gratitude for the people in my life
- being "up for the challenge"!

Not once did I mention my weight or size—just the freedom that comes when I nurture my body and mind. Take a moment to jot down what health feels like to you. See page 151 in the Appendix.

Just as it is important to pinpoint the awesome gifts of health, we can be equally motivated to act in order to *avoid* negative emotions and feelings. Remember how painful it can be when we allow ego threats to bully us? When we fail to make empowering choices, ones that are not in our best interest, how do we feel?

Although this may not be the most pleasurable list to create, identifying the negative emotions that we want to avoid is extremely motivating. When we fail to treat ourselves with love and respect, it is vital to identify the negative experiences for which we are *alone* responsible. Again, I have included my personal list of the feelings or experiences that emerge when I have not chosen to honor my body, mind, or spirit. I can look at this list time and again to remind myself why I choose to take care of myself—especially when I may not feel like it.

QUESTION TWO: What experiences or feelings emerge when you fail to take care of your health?

Here is my personal list:

- disheartened
- worried
- tired
- colorless
- bloated
- apathetic
- stressed over little details
- disconnected from my clothes and body
- cold
- stale taste in my mouth
- angered by small things
- discomfort in my stomach
- critical and judgmental of others
- lonely
- lacking gratitude
- irritated
- hostile and uncompassionate toward strangers
- rushed
- not even attempting to dream "big"
- restless
- limited by anything and everything
- tired, sore eyes
- dull skin

- ignoring my gut feeling
- procrastinating
- eating foods to satisfy boredom
- simply existing
- wasting time
- eating chemically laden, nutritionally dead foods
- feeling invisible
- being hungover
- self-disgust
- depression
- dieting and constantly thinking about food

When our motivation wanes and we don't *feel* like remaining committed to our health goals, having clarity on how certain choices make us feel is crucial to motivating better choices. No one else is better equipped to know what motivates us than ourselves! However, if we believe that changing our current habits will be *more painful* than experiencing these unpleasant feelings, we will not venture to try. This is why your list is so important—it must "hit home." In order to motivate better choices, we must feel compelled to avoid these painful consequences.

How Can I Use My Intrinsic Motivators to Make Better Choices?

In facing life's challenges, including weight loss, we can turn to these powerful feelings to encourage us throughout our lifetimes. The next time that you feel challenged, indecisive, frustrated, upset, or confused, take a deep breath, relax, and refer to your list of emotions and ask:

"Will this action I am about to take make me feel *empowered*?" (or joyous, or proud, or healthy, or so on)

"How can I react to this situation in order to experience *happiness*?" (or optimism, or appreciation, or gratitude, or so on)

In order to avoid painful feelings, ask yourself:

"If I continue with this behavior, am I going to feel *guilty* later on?" (or angry, or ashamed, or depressed, or so on)

At first it may feel calculated to have to "check in" on your feelings *but it is here, at the level of feeling, where we begin to expand our consciousness.* Slow down, become aware of the voice inside you that urges you to love, grow, and express your authentic self. It is always worth the effort to question habitual reactions and behaviors in an attempt to experience our true selves. By referring to our lists of what intrinsically motivates us, we can more easily choose wellness over immediate gratification. We are beginning to create a foolproof plan.

QUESTION THREE: Do you want to feel freedom?

What obstacles or actions are stopping you from experiencing your "healthy and fit" list right now? When you look at your list of "unhealthy" experiences, are you okay with feeling this way? Who or what is stopping you from feeling free? Are you content to continue living in this manner?

Be conscious of your answers to these questions. Review them often until they are a part of your daily thinking. You are now in an excellent place to begin a *conscious journey* toward health and weight loss. There is nothing outside of you more powerful than what you already carry in your heart. The only quick fix I have ever discovered is at the core of these answers. They will offer you strength and clarity when you need it most. Honor this list and connect with the greatest motivational short cut to realizing your goals.

CHAPTER SEVEN

Soul Food—for a *Whole* Life

O NCE WE HAVE uncovered our intrinsic motivators—the true desires of our hearts—we still need an
action-based guide to bridge the gap between intention and
reality. This bridge allows us to *experience* our true essence.

Many of our lives are moving at such a rapid pace that
too often we neglect to make time for personal pleasure;
those daily activities that replenish our spirit and bring joy
to our lives. Unfortunately, when most of us ask, "What
do I *really need* right now?" it's an entirely foreign question, drawing a blank, glazed expression in response. Feeding the soul is about acting "self-fully" (never to be
confused with selfishly); refilling the day with activities that
provide "soul" rewards: pleasure, creativity, relaxation, inspiration, personal empowerment, a sense of mastery, and
love, to name a few.

Although we may desire similar soul rewards, we are all unique in how or where we find them. My two closest friends have very different tastes and hobbies, yet they both share a deep respect for the same soul rewards. Paula finds it incredibly exciting to speak in front of large audiences. Her best qualities come forth while speaking publicly. She feels empowered for hours after giving a speech. Steff, on the other hand, dislikes anything remotely related to public speaking. She once told me that she would rather suffer through a root canal than give a speech. We all have different tastes. Although *you* may find something rewarding, it may not be rewarding for someone else. It is not for us to judge what others find soul-fulfilling. As we allow others (and this means everyone: family, lovers, friends, and coworkers) to walk their paths, we, too, are free to consciously choose our own soul food without reservation or apology.

Becoming comfortable with our uniqueness is a blessing, yet we must also deal with the fact that our interests change. Change is the exciting and beautiful opportunity to create, again and again, how we want to feel in life. Our soul food, therefore, is not always constant. Some things will nurture us throughout a lifetime while others are temporary interests that serve us for only a brief period. Nevertheless, anything that reminds us of our spiritual self has value.

Nurturing our souls connects us to our spirits

The desire to lose weight is only one aspect of your life, yet to be successful in any one area, we must nurture the whole. This next exercise focuses on your entire life—your wholeness—helping you to reconnect with your authentic self. As you gather your soul food ingredients, keep one thing in mind—YOU. All of this is about *you*. About *your* fulfillment. It is not about what you think you should do, enjoy, or create, but instead, what is in your heart, aching to get out.

Start by thinking about the times in your life when you felt carefree, deeply connected, lost in the moment, energized, and happy to be alive. What were you doing? Do these actions or experiences continue to produce these feelings? If so, then include them in your current list. If not, what activities today create those same feelings? Take some time to let those feelings surface. What actions or behaviors are they attached to?

To help you flesh out your ideas, I have included a list of empowering emotions—our intrinsic motivators. Try to focus on a certain emotion and see if you can remember what you were doing when you last experienced this feeling. Start with just one or two emotions and write freely.

For example: If I focus on the feeling of "competence," the first thought that comes to mind is running the Vancouver Sun Run last April, an annual ten-kilometer race. It was a fresh spring morning. All I could see were brightly colored balloons and thousands of people smiling and cheering. My body was relaxed, my face hot, and as I crossed the finish line, a proud voice inside my head said, "You did it. Good work." As I remember this moment, other "competent" memories start to jump into my head:

getting my driver's license; graduation day at university; getting my first article published; traveling through Australia on my own; the first time I prepared a Mother's Day brunch for eight people—what a hit!

Pick a *motivator* to reflect on:

Intrinsic motivators:

Freedom, excitement, joy, effortlessness, peace, gratitude, love, competence, creativity, serenity, elation, empowerment, bliss, inspiration, connectedness, happiness. Add to these as you please.

Exercise #4
Soul Food

This exercise is intended to help you reconnect with the things that add joy and passion to your life. I have provided some brainstorming suggestions to help you get started. Some of these suggestions may apply to you, some may not. See page 154 in the Appendix.

· List the items or activities that make you feel cared for.

· What makes you laugh? What makes you feel silly and carefree? In whose company do you feel happy?

· How do you relax?

· What makes you feel attractive?

- What do you do that contributes to a good day at work?

- Look around the surroundings in your home. What do you enjoy about your residence? How can you create more pleasure where you live?

- What are you interested in learning about?

- What do you want to improve or develop in yourself, your community, or your world?

- What do you enjoy doing with your partner, your friends, your parents, your children? How do you nurture your loved ones?

- Ultimately, what do you desire in your life?

Please add your own individual ideas to your recipe as this list is just a start. The more personal your recipe, the more flavorful the result. *Bon appétit!*

You may find yourself asking, "But my goal is weight loss. How can beautifying my home, laughing with friends, or meditating help me lose weight?"

Expressing ourselves in everything that we do is inextricably linked to losing weight. This is an important point. Taking action daily to create feelings of empowerment, joy, freedom, acceptance, and peace is the first step to getting back to our true self.

For example, by beautifying and organizing our home we are making a statement about our *inner* home. We are expressing that orderliness, balance, and beauty are important in our lives. This spills over into how we view our body and ourselves. As we get rid of the clutter and junk that we no longer use, we become open to discarding dated beliefs that interfere with losing weight. All of these little messages greatly affect our overall consciousness, helping to support our specific weight loss plan, while improving our lives in general. By participating in actions and behaviors that create empowering emotions, we are expressing the deepest thoughts and feelings about *who we really are.* Nurturing *all* areas of our lives gives us the strength to honor our health and fitness goals.

Our Soul Food Helps Us Create Our Own Reality

With each new interaction we share with another person, with every bite of food that we willingly eat, with every thought we *choose* to have about our body, we have the ability to create our experiences. Although we may not have control of how situations unfold or how others react, we do have absolute control of how we choose to feel about it. In fact, we are *responsible* for how we choose to feel about our lives.

I hope you have just spent a substantial amount of time creating lists. Consider how few people make the effort to actually define what brings them pleasure or to question what it is they truly desire. Congratulate yourself! You have just completed the hardest part of the journey. Having been in your shoes, I am excited for the gifts that await you.

Those who seek the desires of their heart will be rewarded. Have faith.

Over the next few days, simply get acquainted with your lists. Later on, we will be combining these lists with others in order to create your own personal daily plan for lifelong health and happiness.

CHAPTER EIGHT

The Natural Truth—Eating for Health and Weight Loss

IF YOU HAVE skipped the first seven chapters looking for the diet portion of this book, I am happy to have caught you now in order to restate the message of the former chapters. Figuring out what to eat has always been a *secondary* issue in the weight-loss quest. Our primary goal is to first rediscover our true essence so that we may live our lives *on purpose*. From a spiritual perspective, our purpose in life is to creatively express our inherent state of joy, freedom, happiness, abundance, compassion, and love.

When we are honoring our physical health, we are simultaneously expressing our spirit. If you can accept this belief as your own, then you will agree that the body does not *confine* the soul, but *expresses* it. Previous chapters covered this principle extensively, which leads us to Chapter Eight, the simplest part of our quest. If we want to experience optimal health and well-being, what are some basic guidelines for healthy eating?

How Does Your Body Want to Feel?

We sometimes eat foods that may be pleasurable going down, but our digestive systems ache and churn for sympathy moments later, yet, despite these physical maladies, we continue. We drink one too many glasses of wine and suffer through a wicked headache twelve hours later, even though our bodies gave us ample warning that we should have stopped at glass number three. We pin ourselves to chairs, gazing at computer screens or televisions for hours, although our bodies are grateful when we stand up, stretch, and take a deep breath. Wouldn't we find it inspiring if our bodies could actually voice their opinions on our health? Well, they do—all the time. We just choose to intercept their intelligent whispers and ignore our bodies' precious feedback.

For a moment, stop and focus on your body. Imagine your heart beating, enzymes digesting, cells repairing, and blood circulating. The body's intelligence is constantly communicating as it performs infinite interactions in order to maintain its homeostasis and health. As you sit comfortably, reading these words, your body is continuously working in order to maintain your survival.

Imagine what the body must endure on a daily basis: pollution, suboptimal foods, inactivity, stress, and chemicals, to name a few. What simple ingredients does your body really need in order to experience optimal health? Fresh air to breathe, pure water, cell-enriching foods, restful sleep, and movement. These are the body's simple and natural needs. How can we lighten the workload for our system so that we may experience the energy and effortlessness of a healthier body? What has distracted us from a natural state of physical well-being?

We Are Living in Weight-Challenged Times

Today's culture is full of time- and money-saving solutions intended to increase our productivity and overall life satisfaction. Unfortunately, most of these solutions are big obstacles to our health and weight loss efforts. We live in a world of fast-food restaurants. The ability to super-size meals and drinks is not only widely available but relatively inexpensive, too. There are thousands of processed, denatured, genetically engineered foods that didn't even exist on supermarket shelves fifteen years ago, many of whose long-term effects on our health are still unknown. Eating away from the home is now a daily occurrence. There is an endless supply of passive entertainment to lull us into a sedentary state. The number of obesity-reducing drugs is on the rise. Plastic surgery quick-fixes are becoming fashionable. As these trends continue, what beliefs do they foster in our lives? Do you subscribe to either of these two attitudes?

1. We can—and should—be immediately gratified.

· Buying prepared and precooked food is less time-consuming and overwhelmingly available. Caught up in our busy lives, we opt for quick and easy foods for both snacking and entire family meals. Laden with salt, sugar, saturated fats, chemicals, and preservatives, these foods save time and provide instant pleasure. Although the nutritional value of these foods is marginal, we compromise our health in order to stay "caught up in the busy-ness."

· It is often more economical to go for the bigger version when eating out. For only "89¢" extra you can order the "combo deal" and in doing so, double the calories you consume. This is not only happening in fast-food establishments—many casual restaurants offer extra food for a nominal fee. Don't buy into it. Why do we need thirty-six ounces of cola? Entire meals have become "bottomless." Our bodies have become habituated to huge amounts of food. We have lost the connection between portion size, our appetites, and healthy satiety. There is no end to our consumption of massive quantities of food as long as we are ordering for *quantity* based on *value*.

2. We can have it all.

Or, more appropriately, we are enticed to *want* it all. Technology has landed us in a strange predicament. We are able to explore the entire world within minutes as we sit in front of our computers, still wearing our pajamas. There is less waiting for *everything* today. Don't like your nose, receding hairline, or gender? Fine, change it! Today's woman is told that she can and should *have it all* in every area of her life. A satisfying career, a loving, romantic relationship, a fit body, an attractive home, well-behaved, happy children, and the list continues.

If we turn our focus to weight loss, is it true that we can have our cake, eat it all, and reach our fitness goals? No. It is simply a lie; we cannot have it all. We cannot sit on our couches night after night for years, feeding ourselves nutrient-poor, calorie-dense foods, and expect to experience optimal well-being. We cannot feed our minds with messages that undermine our worthiness and expect to have peace of mind and fulfillment, nor can we believe that, by losing weight alone, our entire lives will be easy and problem-free.

When it comes to our weight-loss lifestyles, we simply cannot have *everything*. The choice and responsibility is placed in our capable hands. This *not having it all* is actually positive—liberating. Not having it all translates into having a little bit of everything, which leads to balance, and as we begin to define what our own personal balance is, we begin to walk the path of health.

Eating . . . for All the Right Reasons

Next to death and taxes, eating takes a close third on the list of things in life that we cannot avoid—and why would we want to? Unlike the first two, eating is one of life's greatest pleasures. We know that overindulging and gorging will not lead us to health, just as we know that deprivation will not, either. Although we may have tried both routes, neither path has likely led us to our destination. Can we agree then, once and for all, that dieting is not an option?

The Final Word on Dieting—The Ultimate Punishment

We all know that short-term, restrictive diets are negative experiences, but beyond our own trials and tribulations, what do other struggling dieters teach us? As a nation, we are willing to spend billions of dollars annually on diet aids proving our desire to shed extra pounds. But we continue to gain *more* weight year after weight-loss-obsessed year. The nation's population of overweight individuals is now estimated at sixty-one percent. About one-third are obese, meaning that they are 20 percent above normal, healthy weight. Do you believe that we would have such an epidemic on our hands if dieting (by the popular definition of restricting food regardless of hunger) was actually pleasurable?

When we diet, often our entire focus is food. The lack of it, the abundance consumed last night, the good foods, the bad foods, and the all-consuming thought that "Yesterday I beat food, today it beat me. Maybe tomorrow I'll have another chance." This is not healthy, nor is it empowering. It is punishment, clear and simple.

When we diet, we ignore the body's signals of hunger and fullness and, instead, decide randomly what we will and will not eat. Many diets support avoiding entire groups of foods—like carbohydrates! Anyone who has ever cut out all carbohydrates or all fats from their diet for any length of time, knows that it makes them more interested in food—sometimes to the exclusion of anything else. This is punishment. Most likely, some weight will be lost, yet the torment of avoiding the foods we love is usually not offset by the joy we derive from losing a few pounds. Eventually we break the diets and eat these "outlawed" foods anyway. What emotions follow? Disappointment. Guilt. Frustration. These are the very emotions we wanted to avoid. Look at the common response we have when we fail our diets: "I will try harder (to deprive myself) tomorrow." What does this amount to? That's right, more punishment.

Studies have shown that when we break our diets repeatedly, 95 to 98 percent of us will end up regaining all of the weight we lost and more—another blow to our self-esteem. Our dieting failures cannot be attributed to a lack of willpower. Feeling deprived and hungry simply doesn't intrinsically motivate us; in fact, it is the ultimate punishment. We are just trying to avoid pain, as we naturally should. Say "no" to punishment by saying "no" to restrictive diets.

An Integrative Approach to Eating

As the philosophical Buddhists would propose, enlightenment, as well as health, is found through the Middle Path. Balance. Yet, again, we run into trouble. We are all so different. Balance to one may be very different to another. How can we find a diet that works for everyone? We can't, but we can look beyond trendy diets and quick fixes to uncover a holistic, integrative approach to eating that will feed mind, body, and spirit.

- Choose foods for both pleasure and health; they are not mutually exclusive.

- Eat foods that you enjoy, both for taste and texture—don't eat foods that you don't like, even in the name of health—there are many healthy choices available that you can enjoy.

- Eat enough to satisfy hunger, but stop prior to feeling uncomfortable or sluggish.

- Take time to enjoy meals. Many of us spend all day consumed by thoughts of food or eating, yet devour our food within minutes. Instead, engage your mind on what you are doing throughout the day and, come mealtime, be attentive to the food that you are eating, savoring flavors and appreciating its source.

- Eat from a varied selection of foods, including most or all of the food groups (discussed later on in this chapter).

- Never indefinitely swear off eating your favorite foods. In fact, plan to enjoy them once in a while.

- Pay attention to how certain foods make you feel. If you like the taste of creamy, rich foods but later you feel sluggish and have a hard time digesting that food, take note. Your body is giving you important feedback. Likewise, be conscious of the foods that seem to increase your appetite as you eat them. What foods do you find difficult to stop eating even after you are no longer hungry? Try to recognize which foods give you instant gratification but lingering pain later. Becoming more aware of the body's intelligence empowers you to make better food choices.

- Let your body decide when it's time to eat, not the clock. Allow your body to take control of its appetite. You may not be ready for breakfast until 10:00 A.M. instead of 8:00 A.M., or maybe your body prefers to eat an early dinner at 5:00 P.M. instead of waiting until 7:30 P.M. If you are hungry at 4:00 P.M., don't wait until the next socially acceptable mealtime to satisfy your body's needs. Skip the snack foods (which can often be high in fat, sugar, and salt) and instead have a balanced, satisfying meal. Chances are, you will only want to eat something light in the evening.

Eating, Enjoying, and Losing

When it comes to discussing food with my clients, I am always prepared for one particular question. It is prefaced with "Can I eat . . ." and is completed with any item ranging from almonds to fried zucchini sticks. Everywhere we turn, we are being told what to eat or not to eat, so I *do* understand where this question is coming from, and it is valid, as most of us just want clarity on what is considered healthy or unhealthy food. However, I have had many clients who understood, perfectly well, the foundations of a healthy diet, yet whose approach toward food was a constant negotiation of what they could "get away with eating, and still lose weight." Since I don't believe in outlawing any one food, my response was always, "of course you can eat it, once in a while." Happy with the response, we'd continue. Minutes later my client would ask, "Deb, how much of *this* can I eat . . . ?" and I'd soon realize that they were happy to give up responsibility, in a way, hoping that I would prescribe a diet—the very thing we are all trying to get away from!

It's tricky to try to explain to these individuals that their attitude toward weight loss is once again going to renew their membership to the "Diet Club" faster than they can say "Krispy Kreme doughnut." Getting advice from a personal trainer, nutritionist, or doctor does not negate personal responsibility or common sense. As long as these clients tried to find ways around eating a diet primarily based on natural, unrefined foods, it would only be a matter of time before they entertained the thought of another quick-fix plan.

How can we lighten the workload for our system so that we may experience the energy and effortlessness of a healthier body?

With good intentions, we may be trying to lose weight by eating foods that are marketed to us as appropriate "diet" choices. The colorful packaging and catchy commercials push these low-fat items into our grocery baskets, and nature has a hard time competing for our attention. However, many of these low-fat foods are highly processed, chemically laden, and nutritionally vacant. If we begin to think of our diets as a way to feed our cells with life-enriching fuel, we are making huge mistakes by choosing diet foods to get our engines revving. In fact, most of us will run out of gas before we can even lace up our running shoes.

High-Performance Fuel

When choosing foods for health and well-being, simple is better. The more often you choose unrefined, natural foods over processed, manufactured food "creations," the more life you are putting back into your body's engine. Portion size is a factor in controlling weight, but as we begin to fill up with nutrient-rich, fiber-dense, water-packed natural foods, wonderful health benefits follow: our appetites and blood-sugar levels stabilize, our energy levels surge, our moods improve, and our needs for excessive amounts of food decrease. Our bodies' whispers rise to roars!

I have outlined six guidelines for choosing foods that provide the body and mind with "high performance" fuel. I follow these guidelines myself, as much as I possibly can, which I estimate is about 85 percent of the time. It works for me. Many of my clients who have been open to choosing food for its *élan vital,* or life force, have also benefited greatly—benefits that go far beyond just losing weight.

Six Guidelines for Empowered Eating

1. Choose fresh, whole foods in their natural states, free from pesticides, preservatives, or additives

- If we are going to start eating to live, we must start eating *live* foods. Live foods, such as fruits and vegetables, have high amounts of readily available, naturally balanced nutrients. These foods require minimal energy to digest.

- Try organic or locally grown produce for both health and flavor. It is becoming increasingly easier to buy foods in their unaltered and uncontaminated state. Organic vegetables, fruits, grains, and beans that were once found only in specialty stores can now be purchased at local supermarkets.

- Choose poultry, meat, fish, eggs, and dairy raised in their natural environments. Ask for "free-range," "free-run," "organically fed," and "Born 3" items.

- When shopping for packaged items, read labels beyond calories and fat grams. Avoid foods with MSG, chemical sweeteners, food dyes, and other chemical additives and preservatives. Our body recognizes and thrives on natural, real food. We were not designed to ingest so many foreign chemicals. Make purity the priority.

But with all of these suggestions, even small changes can make a difference. I am not suggesting that you become adamant about eating only organic products or become afraid to eat anything that you don't prepare yourself. Remain flexible. Do the best you can. Even though I do buy organic produce, I still frequently eat out. I may not always be able to get a perfect meal, but if I keep health in mind, rarely do I have difficulty ordering a nutritious meal. As you make the effort to seek out high-quality, cell-enriching foods, the taste alone will motivate you to purchase and prepare them.

2. Reduce white flour and white sugar

White flour and white sugar are so refined and processed that they are called "empty calories" for a good reason. There is nothing nutritionally valuable about these two food items, yet they still dominate most contemporary diets today. Although white flour and white sugar are two sources of carbohydrates, we get into trouble when we lump all carbohydrates into the same empty pot. Many trendy diets are cashing in by pushing diets that limit or ban carbohydrates for weight loss, yet how can we justify comparing a carrot to a can of soda?

We need to eat carbohydrates to be healthy—it is the body's preferred energy source, so before you start memorizing the glycemic index[1] of foods and eliminating certain life-giving fruits and vegetables from your diet, use common sense. Doughnuts, white bread, candy, pastries, soda— these foods are the problem, not the whole grains, fruits, vegetables, beans, and lentils in our diet. *If we got rid of the white flour and white sugar in our diets we would eliminate almost all of the health- and weight-loss–related problems associated with eating carbohydrates.*

Years ago, when I was sick, I had been eating a diet consisting primarily of sugar and white flour products. I experienced both physiological and emotional damage from eating these empty foods. An average day of eating used to look like this:

---

[1]The GI is simply a rating of carbohydrates or sugars based on how quickly your body digests them. If you digest them quickly, they are likely to push your blood sugar levels up dramatically and thus force the release of insulin, leading to increased fat storage. This rating does not account for the nutritional value of a food and is therefore an incomplete way to determine which foods are worth consuming.

Food Item:	*Primarily consists of:*
Breakfast: coffee with milk and sugar	*(sugar)*
toast and jam—two slices	*(white flour and sugar)*
Lunch: saltine crackers, 10 to 12	*(white flour)*
a banana or orange	
Diet Coke	*(chemical sweetener)*
Snack: bag of low-fat pretzels	*(white flour)*
Dinner: two cups of pasta with canned pasta sauce	*(white flour/sugar in sauce)*
commercial soft-serve frozen yogurt	*(high in sugar)*

When I took an honest look at my daily food choices, they were almost entirely made of flour and sugar! I thought I was doing a fairly good job, but I was not even close. I felt horrible and the only thing I was losing was my mind. Although my fat intake was marginal, I was lacking the essential fatty acids needed for a healthy functioning metabolism. My vitamin, mineral, fiber, and protein intakes were totally insufficient. My moods were all over the place, my body was either revved up or listless, and my cravings for more of the same dead foods grew. Why?

When we eat white flour and white sugar we do not feel satiated; in fact, our appetites often increase due to our high blood sugar and insulin levels. Cakes, pastries, donuts, cookies, packaged breakfast cereals, and most commercial muffins are particularly addicting because they contain both white flour and white sugar—a double whammy. I was unaware that these foods caused irritability, mood swings, nervousness, and other forms of emotional and physical imbalance. Eating these "dead foods" undoubtedly played a large role in the progression of my eating disorder. As I recognized that white flour and sugar were obstacles to my recovery, I began to make small changes. For example, I began to buy unrefined, preservative-free breads from a bakery. Flaxseed, cracked wheat, and whole-grain rye are still my favorites. I began to use sugar-free jams and apple butters on my toast. For snacks, I replaced floury pretzels with fruit and yogurt, or a slice of rye bread with turkey. Including protein sources with each meal or snack helped stabilize my blood sugar and I noticed that my cravings for "a hit of the white stuff" decreased. For dinner I focused on color (broccoli, yams, yellow and red peppers, etc.) paired with salmon, tuna, chicken, or a hearty vegetable soup. White flour and sugar were not only destroying my health but were also taking the place of foods that I needed to restore it. *As you reduce white flour and sugar in your diet, you will improve your health immediately.*

If you have been eating a diet high in refined flours and sugars, you may find it challenging to even *reduce* your consumption of these foods. Therefore if you want to wean yourself off sugar, start by choosing items that are sweetened with more natural products like stevia, brown rice sweetener, or fruit juice. If your supermarket doesn't carry healthy dessert alternatives, check your local health-food store. Again, read labels and look for hidden sugars as they are often found in the packaged foods that you may least suspect. (Anything that ends in "-ose" is a simple sugar. This includes sucrose, glucose, maltose, lactose, fructose—also, honey and molasses are refined sugars.) Remember, these items are still dessert choices and not staple foods. Just because you buy them from a health-food store doesn't mean that they can be eaten without using common sense.

3. Cooking methods

Any form of cooking begins to destroy the potential nutrient value of food. Do not overcook fruits, vegetables, meats, fish, or poultry.

- Lean toward steamed, baked, poached, grilled, or roasted foods. Reduce food that is fried or microwaved. These choices will help to minimize the destruction of nutrients and retain more of the food's natural water content.

- Try to avoid food descriptions such as Alfredo, au gratin, bearnaise, tempura, breaded, escalloped, creamy, crispy, flaky, Hollandaise, puffed, or battered. These terms primarily refer to foods prepared with a high amount of added fat.

4. Get enough protein

Protein is essential for growth and development. It provides the body with energy and is needed for the manufacture of hormones, antibodies, enzymes, and tissues. Many women dieters often eliminate protein from their diets in an attempt to reduce fat. However, if a woman is deficient in *essential*[2] amino acids, the building of protein in the body stops and the body suffers. Muscles are the fat-burning engines that keep our metabolism high. We need our muscles to help develop a strong, lean body. Including sources of protein in our daily eating plan helps keep our muscles from atrophy and deterioration.

· Choose lean, good-quality meats, fish, and poultry. Do not overcook protein sources as the quality and availability of protein decreases as it is increasingly denatured.

· Vegetarians should ensure protein consumption is complete by learning how to properly combine beans with nuts, brown rice, seeds, corn, and wheat. www.vrg.org is a great vegetarian web site. (It is listed in the Resources section on page 171 along with other healthy, informative, and inspiring sites.)

---

[2]*Essential* amino acids: the body cannot synthesize certain amino acids, and therefore must obtain them from the diet.

Eating small quantities of protein throughout the day helps reduce sugar cravings.

- Try to include a glass of skim milk or an egg at breakfast.

- Snack on low-fat yogurt with fruit.

- Use a good quality whey-protein powder. It's quick, easy to use, and can travel with you in powder form until you need to use it. I put it in my morning smoothie (one scoop of whey-protein, fresh fruit, a tablespoon of flaxseed oil or flaxseeds, and water). Not only is it delicious, but it also has all the energy and nutrition that my body needs until lunch.

- Eat low-fat cottage cheese, which is packed with protein.

- Put a few slices of good quality deli-style meat, chicken, or turkey on high-fiber, low-fat crackers. I enjoy different kinds of mustards with this snack. Discover a flavor that you enjoy.

- Experiment with some of the protein bars on the market. Although I would prefer to eat a proper meal, sometimes it's just not possible. Having a good-quality protein bar in my bag has saved me many times from grabbing something unhealthy while on the run.

Try some of these suggestions and see if your cravings for nutritionally poor foods diminish.

5. Choose good fats, eliminate the rest

Fatty acids are the basic building blocks of which fats and oils are composed. We need fat, but not the type or quantity that we primarily eat in our diets. The fatty acids that are necessary for health and that cannot be made by the body are called *essential fatty acids* (EFAs). They are sometimes also referred to as polyunsaturates or vitamin K. EFAs improve skin and hair, reduce blood pressure, aid memory, and reduce blood clot formation. They also make our food taste more flavorful, helping to satisfy our appetites.

The omega-3 and omega-6 oils are the two essential fatty acids found in fish, raw nuts, seeds, legumes, primrose oil, sesame oil, soybean oil, grapeseed oil, fish oil, flaxseed oil, and certain vegetable oils. Not only do these fats keep skin feeling supple, but they also act as natural anti-inflammatories for joints. We could safely eliminate all other forms of fat in our diets and maintain optimal health by regularly ingesting these essential fats. In fact, craving fatty foods may be a sign that your body is deficient in these two EFAs.

Essential fatty acids are destroyed when heated, so use these oils in salad dressings, in blended drinks, brushed on vegetables and fish after they have been cooked, or drizzled on rice or pasta.

6. Clean water

Drink pure, uncontaminated water. You have probably heard this before and for a good reason: water is an essential nutrient that is involved in every function of the body. Over 70 percent of the body is water. This important fluid transports nutrients and waste products in and out of cells. It is necessary for all digestive, absorption, circulatory, and excretory functions. It is also necessary for maintaining proper body temperature and utilizing water-soluble vitamins.

Each function that water performs in our body aids healthy weight loss. Try to drink a substantial amount of pure water each day (six 8-ounce glasses is a good guideline but increase consumption before, during, and after exercise, especially in warm weather).

· Avoid caffeine and carbonated beverages. Opt for fresh-squeezed juices, herbal teas, or natural coffee substitutes like *Caf-Lib* (www.caf-lib.com). Try drinking hot water with fresh ginger slices throughout the day—it is both cleansing and good for digestion.

Quite often we crave salty and sugary foods when in fact our body may actually be in the initial stages of dehydration.

· When you wake in the morning your body has gone for over eight hours without any fluid. Place a glass of water beside your bed at night and drink it first thing in the morning to rehydrate your system. In a few days, it will begin to taste better on your empty stomach than coffee ever could.

· At work, try keeping a large bottle of water beside your desk, drinking two-thirds to one cup of water every hour, refilling as needed.

Make It Personal

When it comes to choosing a style of eating, beyond anything else, it needs to suit *your style*. There are many healthy methods to eat and lose weight (both carnivores and vegetarians enjoy good health), but, ultimately, you must be comfortable and satisfied to adopt an eating style that can last you a lifetime. I hope you are open to these nutritional suggestions, but as I have clearly stated throughout this book, *ultimately it is you who must decide how to use this information*. What makes sense to you? What "speaks" to you? What are you willing to experiment with?

If you do choose to experiment with the guidelines presented here, make small changes, one at a time. Get comfortable with the change before you implement a new guideline. Often our taste buds have been so vandalized by the high content of salt and sugar in our foods that vegetables and fruits may, at first, seem bitter or unappealing. As you clean up your palate, the delicious taste of fruits and vegetables will return. Today, a luscious papaya tastes more blissfully sweet and satisfying to me than any over-processed white cake. Be patient, *it will happen.*

I review this list regularly to see where I can improve my own eating style. I have found it very helpful to learn as much as I can about nutrition. It has given me the knowledge and tools to fine-tune my own style of eating to suit my particular preferences. Both the library and bookstore carry many recipe books that support these guidelines. (See also the Resources section on page 169 for additional information.)

As we begin to incorporate healthier food choices into our day-to-day routines, we rebuild foundations—not only of health but also of empowerment—and the weight begins to come off.

How Do We Stop Food Cravings?

Trying to stick to a restrictive diet is one of the fastest ways to start craving *everything*. The moment my girlfriend tells me she is going on a ten-day juice diet, I start craving food for *her*—particularly when I notice her hungry eyes coveting my turkey sandwich.

Some researchers speculate that cravings arise in an attempt to supply the body with the nutrients it lacks. If we aren't feeding our bodies with healthy, nutrient-rich foods, cravings serve a purpose—they are nature's way to ensure that our dietary needs get met. In fact, Susan Schiffman, Ph.D., professor of medical psychology at Duke University Medical Center, suggests that carbohydrate cravings can simply be from hunger because our blood sugar levels are too low. Fortunately, when our diet is based on healthy principles versus short-term calorie slashing, most of the physiological reasons for our cravings will be reduced or eliminated.

Emotional cravings are another story. The emotional reasons for our cravings started the moment we entered the world. As infants, the pain and discomfort of hunger was remedied by a bottle, paired with a soft, cozy blanket, a cooing voice, and, minutes later, a full stomach. *Food the comforter*. As children, if we were good, we were given candy or a special treat. *Food the rewarder*. In my house dessert was denied until I finished my most disliked chore—gathering the dirty clothes from where I had un-successfully hidden them under my bed. *Food the negotiator*. Christmas, Easter, Thanksgiving, birthdays, an-niversaries, all good times. *Food the celebrator*. And the dependable liter of Häagen-Dazs in the freezer, always there to catch the tears, as we cried into each spoonful over the sudden loss of our job *and* boyfriend. *Food the friend*.

It's no wonder we have emotional food cravings. We have been taught that eating is an acceptable way to avoid unpleasant emotions and elicit desired ones. Perhaps in many ways it can, yet the consequences of turning to food to feed an emotional or spiritual void has only ever ap-peased us momentarily, in minor ways. The repercussion of emotional eating has brought us far more pain than plea-sure or we wouldn't want to put an end to these powerful cravings!

Unlike physiological food cravings, a balanced meal will not put an end to the emotional cues that trigger overeating. Emotional eating can be a big stumbling block to reaching our fitness and health goals. For many, food is used to help fill an unmet need for fun, excitement, or even love—issues that we all face at one point or another. I would know. I suffered for years, "stuffing" my feelings in an attempt to avoid difficult emotions; yet only when we get in touch with the emotions that drive us toward food do we find freedom from our cravings.

On my road to recovery, in order to resist giving in to cravings and binges, I had to realize that experiencing the urgency and anxiety of the moment was not going to kill me. As uncomfortable and strong as the craving may have been, the most important thing was that I didn't allow myself to eat without awareness. Each time I chose to *feel* the tension instead of giving in to it, I became more empowered. *I could have the impulse to do something destructive to my body and yet not act on it.* What an exciting realization! Here are a few tools to work through when your emotions are telling you that you *need to eat* yet your stomach and common sense are saying that you don't.

1. First ask yourself, "Am I actually hungry?"

Before you condemn yourself for giving in to a few cookies or a handful of chocolate peanuts, trust your body to tell you if you are in fact hungry. Start by having a tall glass of water. Sometimes we mistake dehydration for hunger. Your body may be telling you that you need something, and you assume it's food. Often, rehydrating our systems helps to diminish our cravings.

If you are still unsure whether or not you are hungry, try to do something else for twenty minutes and see if the urge to eat has passed. If you still want something twenty minutes later, chances are you're actually hungry. Energize your body by feeding it a nutrient-dense, healthy meal or snack.

2. If it is not hunger, what am I really feeling?

Try to pinpoint some of the emotions that accompany your moments of weakness. Emotional eaters are often triggered by some of the following feelings:

- Emptiness, loneliness, or a desire for comfort
- Anger, resentment, fear, or frustration
- Stress, tension, anxiety, or insecurity
- Depression or feeling "down"
- Feeling overtired or generally fatigued
- Desire for fun, social activity, or excitement

When the craving hits, take a moment to turn your focus inward and ask, "Is something bothering me, and, if yes, what is it?"

3. Trusting that the negative feeling will pass, can I just BE with this feeling?

In order to resist giving in to cravings and binges, we must realize that experiencing our feelings is the only way that we can start to help ourselves. As powerful as your urge to eat may be, it will pass, and each time that we choose to face the feelings behind the cravings, we become more empowered. If we are unwilling to recognize our loneliness or insecurity, and instead eat through the pain, we cannot fix the problem. In fact, it's just a matter of time before the negative emotions return and we turn to food to numb the emotions.

4. How am I going to feel if I eat this food?

Before you give in to that pizza, ask yourself, "If I eat this right now will I be happy in fifteen minutes? Will eating ten cookies alleviate my feelings of boredom, or will I simply feel angry and frustrated that I overate?" Think ahead to how it feels when you overindulge. Does eating actually make you feel better, or are you simply disappointed and bloated afterward?

5. Is there a better way to take care of myself?

What can you do that will bring you pleasure *and* nurture your body, mind, or spirit? Take a hot bath, phone a friend, write in a journal, get outside for a walk, watch an inspiring movie—take the focus off eating and connect with the things that bring you joy. Turn to your soul-food recipe to find alternate activities that feed your life, not just your stomach.

6. Ask yourself, "What is truly important to me?"

You probably already know that the answer to this question cannot be found in a piece of chocolate cake. So how do you really want to *feel* in your life? After all of the positive things you've done for your health, do you really want to sabotage your efforts by eating through your emotions? Do you want to respect and honor your body, or punish it with bingeing? The choice is yours.

The next time you get an overwhelming craving for an unhealthy food, try to ask yourself these questions first. Chances are you will find better answers looking *within* than you do at the bottom of a bag of Oreos.

Finding Your Ideal Weight

Before we decide what our ideal weights should be, we must first look at the word *ideal*. By definition, "ideal" refers to "conforming to a standard of perfection." Look at the trouble we get into when we interpret this as: "trying to conform to *society's* standard of perfection" as portrayed to us through the media. We need to recognize that the notion of a perfect body or ideal weight is illusory—

varying greatly across cultures. There is no *one* standard of perfection.

Where do we turn to find our ideal weights? We know that we can't rely on the media or the fashion industry to tell us what we should weigh, even though we still get caught in their insidious webs. However, height and weight charts aren't very reliable either, as they are so broad that it's difficult to pinpoint where our unique bodies fit in. We must find a new definition on which to base our ideal weights.

I always *wanted* to weigh 120 pounds. That number was burned into my mind's scale, yet I was making a big mistake by confusing what I *wanted* to weigh with what my *ideal* weight really was. Back then I thought that the two were synonymous. I was wrong. How could a weight be ideal if it meant that I had to physically and mentally starve myself in order to keep the scale from reading "121"? Today I use a different method to discover my ideal weight that may be helpful to you.

My ideal weight is my body's own natural state of perfection.

I don't rely on the media to define how my body should look, nor do I deny my genetics by trying to conform to an unattainable body type or shape. Instead, I honor my genetic makeup, committing to move, feed, and love my body as best I can. When I am living up to my end of the bargain, the number on the scale will reflect my ideal weight.

My ideal weight is the weight at which my body experiences the greatest delight.

When I am at my ideal weight I am released from dieting and obsessive thoughts about food. My body is healthy and fit—free to experience all of my physical desires, like hiking with my dog, wearing clothes that make me feel good, or getting out of the way of a speeding bus! I am able to hear my body's wisdom telling me when to eat and when to stop. My emotions are no longer at the mercy of weight-related issues, affording me the mental energy to pursue the things that bring pleasure to my life. When my weight fluctuates more than five pounds above *or below* my ideal weight, my body always lets me know, as *its delight begins to wane.* Food issues may begin to surface, or perhaps I begin to feel sluggish and uncomfortable in my clothes. I try to remain aware of these clues that tell me when I'm getting off track. It's *my* job to act accordingly in order to restore its balance.

Almost every plan directed at weight loss asks you to state your goal weight. "How much do you want to lose?" It is *the* token question. If you find it motivating to pick a number, a goal weight, and work toward it, then do what works for you. But has this method ever worked for you in the past?

From experience, I feel a far better goal is to take the focus *off* the number that you so eagerly want to see beneath your toes and *reverse* the game. Instead of picking a *goal weight,* why not evaluate your success based on whether or not you have been living up to your end of the bargain? Have you been moving, feeding, and loving your body as best you can? If you can answer "yes," then you are reaching your goal every day. There is no need to weigh yourself, as your body is already moving toward its own natural ideal. Likewise, if you answer "no," then there is still no reason to weigh yourself, as you have other, more important things to do first—like, move, feed, and love your body as best you can. It sounds like double-talk, I know, but I suspect you get the point.

Ultimately, reaching our ideal weights is as much about commitment as it is detachment. It involves a commitment to nurture our souls, to continuously ask, "In what way can I empower my spiritual, emotional, and physical well-being today?" When we make the commitment to ask this question and act on it as best we can, we can remain detached from the number on the scale because we can trust that this commitment *alone* has value, independent of the result. If we are living our lives *on purpose,* we don't need the scale to tell us if we are on track—we'll know it.

CHAPTER NINE

The Real Gifts of Exercise— Exercising Your Right to Enjoyment

EXERCISE IS A key ingredient to living an empowered, healthy life, and although there are literally *hundreds* of very good, scientifically proven reasons to exercise, I am going to refrain from telling you *why* you should do it. Chances are you already know. Instead, I will begin by sharing with you *my* reason for a lifelong commitment to exercise.

Beyond the incredible health and weight-loss benefits of exercise, there is one main reason why I continue to move my body daily, year after year. *It makes me feel incredibly alive.* In fact, through moving and using my body as it was intended, I have experienced every desired emotion from my list of intrinsic motivators. A few examples come to mind immediately.

Joy

If I had to choose one exercise to do for the rest of my life, I'd pick walking. In spite of the copious amount of rainfall in the Pacific Northwest, I always find the motivation to walk, year round. I have *used* walking to soothe my soul, clear my mind, and invigorate my body so many times that I consider it my magic elixir. Walking allows me to tune in to my inside world, while awakening my senses to the simple beauty around me. Walking puts me into this natural, joyous state like no other activity. What activities bring you joy?

Excitement

A healthy dose of competition and challenge adds excitement and fun to our lives. I have tried many sports and although I don't excel in *any* of them, I always enjoy being in a heightened state of emotion and energy. I'm in the moment—concentrating, coordinating, anticipating. Whether I am crossing the finish line of a ten-kilometer race, learning how to smash a tennis ball back at my opponent, or skiing through diamond-sparkling powder, I am experiencing the exhilaration of living. I don't even have to be good at a sport in order to reap the rewards; I just have to be involved. Being active adds immeasurable excitement to my life. Are you able to recognize that being active positively influences your life, far beyond its ability to burn calories?

Love

I schedule time to exercise daily. Some days I go for a long run, on others just a short walk. If I'm feeling tense, I may use the time to stretch. Regardless of what I do, I take the time to do something that is *just for me*. There are times when I am running up a steep hill and I just want to quit, but I encourage myself along, thinking, "just a few more steps," and soon I am at the top, raising my fists into the air for a small victory cheer. What is the message that I am sending to my entire being? *I am worth it*. I am worthy of being loved and taken care of because *I make it so*. We are too ready to give up scheduled exercise, believing that other errands and tasks have much more importance. This is a mistake. We can love the world much better when we love ourselves first. Exercising my body is one of the quickest ways to remind myself that I *matter*.

Exercise engages us in so many ways

These few examples show how we are drawn into life when we are physically participating. I don't feel as if I *have* to exercise. Instead, I *use* exercise in order to feel alive. As I sit and write this sentence, I can feel that my shoulders are beginning to stiffen and my mind is starting to tire. Since I know I need to take a break, I will *use* a walk to rebalance my body and mind. Exercise keeps my physical world connected to my spiritual and emotional

world. There are few things in life that bring me such pleasure. What types of activities do you enjoy?

Making Exercise Pleasurable

Goals give us destinations. It is important to know the
direction in which we are moving and the intended result.
However, if attaining the goal becomes the *only* reason to
exercise, then we are missing the mark. No matter what our
exercise goals are: weight loss, strength, stamina, flexibil-
ity, all of these and more, we will most likely achieve them
as they become secondary to the pleasure of simply participating.

Often, when we only focus on our goals we fail to
listen to our bodies' feedback and end up dropping out,
getting injured, or both. I have made this mistake myself.
After many years of walking for exercise, I began to envy
these gazelle-like creatures effortlessly passing me, their
feet moving swiftly and lightly over the ground. I was inspired to take up running. I set a goal, and with blazing
inspiration, I burned up the pavement. The first few times
that I went running, my legs felt so heavy—as if fresh
concrete had been poured into them—that I hardly made it
down the street before I had to turn around. The moment
I got home, the cement hardened, leaving my lower body
stiff and rigid. I hated it, so I quit, even though my new
shoes were still in showroom condition. I figured that I was
just not cut out to feel like a gazelle.

Three years later I learned to make SMART goals

(goals that are Specific, Measurable, Adaptable, Realistic, and have a Time frame), and I decided to give running a second chance. This time, I allowed myself a full year to become a runner. My main priority was to enjoy each workout pain-free, so that I could look forward to doing it again. In time, I naturally progressed from walking to running. Today, I love running. My heart pounding. Sweat rolling. Ocean air filling my lungs. To me, it is forty-five minutes of indescribable satisfaction, peace of mind, and personal empowerment. And although this may sound like the antithesis of pleasure for you *today*, if you progress at a level that allows you to enjoy each step of the process, you can reach all of your fitness goals and more. As it has been said before, *life is a journey, not a destination*. Therefore, the activities that you choose to participate in should be rewarding, independent of the outcome.

Before you start thinking about where you are headed, think first about your mode of transportation. What activities do you *enjoy* doing? What type of exercise have you enjoyed in the past? What types of activities are you excited about trying? Just like dieting, if you find the activity more punishing than rewarding, you will eventually quit—no matter how easy and fun they make it look in the commercials. List three to five exercise activities that interest you.

How can you reward your efforts? How can you combine exercise with other things you enjoy? The following are some of my own ideas:

- I often exercise with friends. Walking, hiking, roller-blading, skiing, running, going to stretching classes—these are all social activities that you can do with a friend for added enjoyment and encouragement.

- Although I love doing my yoga videotape in my living room, I still go to yoga classes to learn new things and meet like-minded people. It keeps me involved.

- I often plan my exercise around something rewarding. For example, I will plan to walk or jog to my favorite coffee shop where I am rewarded with some quiet time, the daily paper, and a cup of my favorite vanilla-hazelnut tea.

- If you like animals, walk a dog. If you would like to help the environment, bike to work. If you love the ocean, swim, sail, kayak, or windsurf. If you enjoy beautiful gardens, start digging, pulling, and planting. The point is, *make your exercise work for you*.

Become a fan of the activities in which you participate. Find books or magazines devoted to the activity, look up information on the Internet, or see if there are other groups participating in the same activities in your community. There are thousands of books, web sites, groups, events, races, magazines, clinics, and trips devoted entirely to walking. Staying interested and excited about your chosen activity just adds to your success. It may take three months or three years to reach your goals, but if you find a way to enjoy what you're doing, the time it takes won't matter, *and that's what's important.*

If you are starting a new activity or if your fitness level is low, start slowly. Although there will be physical adjustments as you begin any new activity (you'll remember that you *do*, in fact, have muscles), there is no reason why you can't enjoy exercise from day one. I have always taken this approach with my clients. I let *them* decide how hard or fast that they want to go. Safety and enjoyment come first, the details are secondary.

If you are interested in hiring a certified trainer to assist you with your fitness goals, it is a great way to get additional knowledge and learn about safe technique. In fact, by first completing the exercises in this book, you are *guaranteed* to get your money's worth during your sessions. For example, once Renata covered this information, she was able to reap far more benefits from our sessions. Her heart and mind were finally *aligned* with her physical goals.

With or without a trainer, remember to keep *your own personal style* in mind. Be open to trying new things, but if you already know, for instance, that you love the outdoors and don't enjoy exercising around others, there's no point in buying a gym membership. You would be amazed at how many people agree to fitness programs that don't suit their basic interests. Take the time to figure out what works for you, then enjoy yourself.

Creating SMART Goals

Many people start their fitness plans two weeks prior to their tropical beach vacations, and stop them the moment they fasten their seatbelts in preparation for takeoff. Instead of attempting another short-term fitness blitz, guaranteed to leave you discouraged and possibly injured, take some time to create SMART goals that you can use throughout a lifetime. Rather than simply stating, "I want to get more fit," get more specific and detailed about your goal.

Example of SMART *Goal Setting*

Specific   I will learn to jog.

Measurable   I will increase my jogging time by five minutes weekly.

Adaptable   My flu has set me back one week. I will rest this week to avoid more illness.

Realistic   I would like to be able to jog for fifteen minutes without a break.

Time frame   I will reevaluate my goal in two months.

Tips

- Start out by making one or two SMART goals. You can always add more as you go along.

- What does being healthy allow you to do, feel, or experience? Review your list of intrinsic motivators to remind you of why you are doing this.

- Have you explained to family and friends the importance of your goals? In what areas do you need support? The great success of one is almost always owed to many. Asking for assistance is saying, "I am important—I matter."

- When you feel like doing nothing, do a little. Many programs are abandoned because the hour workout seemed overwhelming, so we ended up doing nothing. On days like this, I tell myself, "just five minutes," and if after five minutes I *still* don't want to exercise then my workout is finished. (More often than not, however, once I am moving I feel better and usually continue). *Consistency breeds success.* Doing just ten minutes of exercise consistently is ultimately more important than doing an hour's worth every once in a while.

- Don't be concerned about the fat-burning zone. When trying to burn calories, work as hard as you comfortably can, for as long as you can, remembering that safety and enjoyment come first. The idea that you will only lose fat if you work in some magic "zone" is simply untrue. If you enjoy working at the lower intensities, then you can always burn more energy by going for longer.

- Do not get bogged down in lengthy gym routines and extensive training regimes. As you naturally progress you can increase time, intensity, and frequency of exercise as you need to. The important thing is that you like what you are doing enough to do it consistently.

Refer to page 158 in the Appendix when writing your SMART goals.

Measuring Your Fitness Success Beyond the Scale

Any athlete will tell you that the scale is the *least* helpful measurement in determining fitness level. Here are some great ways to gauge the success of your exercise program, regardless of the scale. If you like, incorporate them into your goals:

1. Resting heart rate

Aerobic activity will lower your heart rate over time, as it reflects your heart's growing strength. Measure your pulse first thing in the morning to accurately record your resting heart rate. Gently place two fingers on the underside of your wrist (where a watchband would rest). For a full minute, count the beats. Every few weeks recount and see if your resting heart rate is dropping.

2. Increased endurance

One of the most inspiring benefits of improving our fitness levels is the increased energy and stamina that we develop as our bodies adapt to their new workload. Wouldn't it be great to have the stamina to put in a full day of work, feed the family, take an hour to yourself for exercise, and *still* be energized to go out for a social evening with friends—on a weeknight? Exercising regularly increases rather than depletes our energy and endurance. See how your day-to-day stamina improves with regular exercise.

3. Count your compliments

When people look at us they first notice the joy, liveliness, and smile on our faces before anything else. In fact, the sizes of our waists are much more noticeable to us than anyone else. As soon as we start to change our attitude toward ourselves, people notice, regardless of weight. Exercising is a great way to reflect our vigor for life, and that is extremely attractive. We feel lighter already. Imagine radiating so much vitality that people couldn't stop telling you about it. Count your compliments in whatever form they come.

4. Clothes size

The changes in body composition due to exercising are often not reflected by the scale. We can lose fat from our thighs and abdomens, gain muscle in our pectorals, and the scale has not moved one bit. However, our shapes have changed, our metabolisms are running like fine-tuned machines, and all of our fitness efforts are paying off. A better way to measure success is to notice how our clothes fit. Within weeks of participating in regular exercise, clothes will start to fit differently regardless of what the scale tells you.

5. *Increased strength*

Just as stamina and energy increase with exercise, so does the ability to open jars, carry luggage, or beat a sister, partner, or son in an arm wrestle. What is getting easier to do in your life? The daily perks of being stronger are both useful and fun, but more important, we also need strength to help protect us from injury and accidents. A fit body is an injury-free body. How are you doing with yours?

6. *Improved sleep*

Adding exercise to our day improves sleep patterns immediately. After an active day, my sleep is more restful and deeper, and I wake up feeling refreshed. Getting adequate rest is crucial to our fitness improvements, as muscle is only built and repaired when we are sleeping. Notice how exercise improves your "night life."

Our journeys toward fitness are a continuous process of renewal and change. When you are ready, take another step on your journey and commit to a safe, *enjoyable* fitness plan the *SMART* way.

CHAPTER TEN

Conscious Living

W HEN I SHARE my story with discouraged clients they often ask me what was *the most important factor* in getting through my food and body-image disorder. Although there are many important facets to recovery, ultimately, I believe my success came from expanding my consciousness—opening my eyes to see the bigger picture of who I really am. As best I could, I refused to fall prey to ego threats. When I no longer measured my worth based on my dress size I was free to become empowered—wired to my intrinsic motivators.

"But how did you open your eyes?" My answer to this question was always incomplete, for I had a hard time explaining such a seemingly personal topic to my clients. I knew that I had experienced a change in my heart, but how did it happen? It was actually sort of a mystery to me, yet after much reflection, I came up with some of the tangible tools that helped me expand my consciousness.

From Reacting to Acting—Taking the First Step

By now I hope that you are comfortable with your list of intrinsic motivators, and understand the value of healthy eating and exercise. These are important tools to your success. But even with the best of intentions we are all apt to get caught off guard—distracted from these tools—and within seconds, we allow self-doubt to seep in, undermining our best intentions. If time and again we are unable to bring our attention back to our purpose, then we fail to change.

Since we are all likely to get sidetracked now and then, how can we train ourselves to remain conscious of our health and fitness goals *in the moment that we are least aware of them*? Here are some suggestions to help increase your level of awareness the moment you get distracted by food, people, or life in general.

Tools for Becoming Instantly Conscious of Goals

· **Take a deep breath.**

As simple as it sounds, this is one of my favorites. Scenario: You are late for work and you can't find your keys. While you are frantically looking for them the phone rings. You rush to pick it up right when the dog starts to bark so loudly that you can't identify the voice on the other end. On your way to work you want to scream, cry, or go to the nearest drive-through food outlet, since you're already late. Instead, breathe! Taking a deep breath is like turning the volume down on the outside world so that you can hear that quiet inner voice urging you to act instead of react.

· **Remove yourself from the situation or the temptation.**

If you feel that a situation is beginning to create too much stress or temptation, remove yourself from the stimulus before you become unaware of your behavior. For example, a superior at work tends to make critical remarks about your performance just prior to your lunch break. Unconsciously you end up soothing yourself with a sugary, refined Danish instead of a nutritious, calming meal. You later recognize that you had eaten out of frustration. Take note. Ask the person if he/she will wait to speak to you after lunch—when you will have already consumed a nutritious meal.

· **Get rid of problem foods.**

Don't be afraid to give or throw away food that you find difficult to stop eating. Do it as soon as you begin to feel overwhelmed.

- **Picture a big STOP sign.**

Big. Red. Powerful. Saving you from a dangerous, distracted moment.

- **Remember a favorite quote and repeat it to yourself.**

By simply repeating a few inspiring words, you can bring your attention back to your goal. I repeat quotes to myself in many situations. Whether I need to be inspired, consoled, encouraged, grateful, or detached from an outcome, there are literally thousands to choose from, found in books or on the Internet. (See the Resources section on page 169.) I have a favorite quote section in my journal so that I can quickly find a suitable quote when I most need it. I have also included a list of empowering and enlightening quotes on pages 163–168.

- **Pick an emotion from your list of intrinsic motivators and imagine experiencing it.**

I have already covered this useful tool in Chapter Six, but it's worth repeating. Every so often I will have a few days where my food choices are based more on circumstances than awareness. Holidays, social events, and stress are just a few obstacles that get in the way of my conscious eating plan. Just last month, for example, I was busier than usual both at work and socially, and found myself eating on the go and in restaurants all week. After a few days of feeling too exhausted to exercise, I realized that I hadn't been eating any vegetables, my water intake had been marginal, and my digestion was sluggish from ingesting more refined food than usual.

Today, after many years of practice, I simply need to remember how inspired and energetic I feel when I eat the foods that feed my cells with life, and that gets me back on track immediately. If you find it difficult to remember how empowered you feel when you are living on track, turn to your *healthy* and *unhealthy* lists to motivate and reinforce better choices.

· **Ask your body how it feels.**

Are you feeling tense from the conversation you just had with your partner? Does your stomach gurgle and bubble after the rich, heavy cream sauce you ate at lunch? Do you feel peaceful and relaxed after a fresh twenty-minute walk? Get "conscious" by turning your attention to how your body is feeling. Are you really hungry—or just tired, thirsty, or mad at your husband? Listen to your body's language. Physically and emotionally, the body speaks the truth. Learn to appreciate its message. It doesn't lie.

· **Place a picture that stirs up positive emotions in a common area of your home or in your wallet.**

If "a picture is worth a thousand words," then choose an image that reminds you of at least a few desired emotions from the list of intrinsic motivators. I have pictures of my beautiful black lab, Justice, throughout the house and although it may sound silly, just catching a glimpse of him is enough to change my mood from that of distracted, bored, or frustrated to one of purity, joy, and love. Pick anything that inspires you: art, nature, a loved one, a picture of a favorite personal memory, and so on. Great places guaranteed to grab your attention: near the bathroom mirror, beside your computer screen, on the fridge, on your desk, and so on.

(For more tips on increasing consciousness and food cravings, see page 92.)

Expanding Overall Consciousness

Troubleshooting obstacles with proven instant solutions is priceless. I still use these simple tools when I need to *slow down* and *get centered* in order to act empowered. But isn't our ultimate goal to be unaffected by these obstacles altogether? The more often we can remain aware of how we are feeling, be attentive to the needs of our body, and remain conscious of the voice that inspires us to love, those pestering moments that challenge our good intentions begin to fade away.

There are so many wonderful ways to develop greater overall consciousness. The following are some of the ways I use to increase daily awareness. Some are short exercises that you can begin practicing today, while others can be life-long ways to increase insight and enlightenment in your life.

· **Listen**

When we begin to truly listen to what is being said around us, what do we notice? What are people really look-ing for? *What do we all want?* Approval, acceptance, ap-preciation, and love? As we practice active listening, we become more aware of the needs around us and, therefore, we are in a better position to give appropriately to others. It takes practice to fully focus on what someone is saying without mentally jumping ahead, planning a response. If we all want to feel accepted and loved, then actively lis-tening to those around us is a great way to nurture the success of a collective goal.

· **Listen to *yourself***

When we speak, how often do we realize that we sound just like one of our parents? Or perhaps our coworkers are constantly making negative comments and we begin to pick up the same habit. Listening to ourselves speak is some-times an unwelcome shock, yet the language that we use characterizes who we are. When we pay close attention to the words coming out of our mouths, do they represent how we truly feel? Do we say what we actually mean? Do our words support our beliefs? Being mindful of our language keeps us aligned with our values and authenticity.

· Silent time

How often do you turn the radio down in the car as you navigate to an unknown destination, or ask people around you to be quiet as you try to recall the name of *that* actress, you know, with the English accent? "Shh, it's on the tip of my tongue." Noise of any kind can distract us from conscious thinking. We need regular moments of silence to help organize our thoughts and feelings. At first, try turning off the radio in the car. Eat a meal without speaking. Turn off the phone. Go for a walk and leave the Sony Walkman at home. Making time for silence helps us naturally sort out the daily input that constantly inundates us.

· Meditation

Voltaire said, "Liberty of thought is the life of the soul." If we want to listen to the voices of our spirits, there is nothing more effective than the daily practice of meditation. There is so much going on in our minds: the daily rush of thoughts, plans, memories, anxieties, and general inner chatter, that even though this inner voice is always present within us, we are often too distracted to recognize it. There are many different forms of meditation, but all aim at freeing the mind of its *usual* thoughts so that a deeper level of consciousness can be experienced.

When people think of meditation they often picture a

seated meditation. This type of meditation may employ visualization or the repetition of a mantra. (A mantra is a sacred chant that has no literal meaning, like *Aummmm*. It is a vibrational sound that, when repeated silently, helps you to reach a more peaceful state of consciousness by interrupting the usual flow of thoughts.)

Practice forms of meditation like Yoga, Tai-chi, and Qi Gong utilize breathing and movement to bring about a sense of harmony and greater unity, but you are not just limited to these forms of movement meditation. There are even simple walking meditations. In fact, when I *run*, I am often centered in the moment, moving rhythmically, using calm, deep breaths, and I experience the same incredible feeling as I do when I practice a seated meditation: a sense of joy and connectedness to all living things.

Although there is a lot of information available regarding how to meditate, do not get overly concerned about whether you are *doing it right* or progressing fast enough. If you want to try a form of seated meditation, start by finding a quiet place to sit, somewhere that you feel comfortable. Close your eyes and relax. Focus your attention on your breathing. When thoughts come into your mind, recognize them without judgment and then simply bring your attention back to your breathing. As your thoughts begin to fade away, you will tap into the spiritual pulse that is constantly present not only in your own body *but throughout the entire universe*. This state is often referred to as "slipping into the gap" or entering the silent spaces between your thoughts. Being restfully alert may be the best way to describe the meditative experience. In these moments we have no memories or desires—we just *are*.

If this state is hard to imagine, think about the experience of when you first wake up in the morning. You are no longer asleep, but you have not yet begun to think about your day ahead or the roles you play as mother, daughter, wife, or so on. You just are. You are ego-free. What silent pleasure! We usually don't realize that we are in this state until we are fully awake. Going into the gap is a similar experience. Don't *try* to experience this state—it won't happen if you do—just relax and settle your mind. Going into the gap is just a benefit of meditating.

At first, try meditating for ten or fifteen minutes during a suitable time. Once you feel comfortable sitting for this amount of time, you can extend your meditation time up to thirty minutes, once or twice daily, if you like.

Meditation has the power to change us profoundly, bringing forth a deeper sense of peace and unity to our lives. When we experience greater wholeness, food becomes powerless—we are complete—and overeating cannot pacify us anymore.

· **Yoga**

Yoga is a system of exercise that consists of a series of poses, postures, and positions. It began in India about five thousand years ago to promote union of mind, body, and spirit. When most people think of yoga they picture the physical aspects, known as *hatha* yoga, which includes various postures or *asanas*. Learning and practicing these postures benefits us physically, but it is the combination of conscious breathing, focused attention, and meditation that make yoga much more than just a form of exercise.

Although there are many great yoga tapes on the market with various styles catering to all levels, you will gain infinitely more by attending a yoga class led by an experienced teacher. The advantage of taking a class is that you will learn proper technique with hands-on assistance. In addition, depending on the teacher, you will be exposed to a greater variety of poses, meditations, chants, and breathing techniques that will expand your experience beyond that of a videotape.

· **Practice being nonjudgmental**

Let go of the need to judge or label things. This includes people, events, and of course, yourself. If we label ourselves as "bad" for overeating, we are unable to see all of the other positive angles and facets of our behavior. We waste a lot of energy this way, yet if we can remain observers we are open to new ideas, change, acceptance, and growth.

Unfortunately, we are all guilty of making snap judgments now and then, with consequences that can often last a lifetime. Think of how limiting this is. Out of laziness and comfort, we are quick to judge, turning away an infinite number of other options and possibilities. The next time that you feel like passing judgment, see if you can turn the situation around. Can you see the person or situation from a different point of view? When we cease to judge and label the people we encounter, we become more compassionate and understanding of others, and by not judging others, we free ourselves from self-judgment.

· **Adopt an attitude of gratitude**

We are so quick to judge and condemn our bodies that we are rarely grateful for the miraculous feats that they accomplish day after day. Infants are born with fatal diseases, many wheelchair-bound children will never have the experience of running on a grassy field, and millions of people rely on medications (with unpleasant side effects) in order to remain alive. There are people dying of illnesses all around us and although these facts are incredibly disheartening, I encourage you to adopt an *attitude of gratitude* for your body, for the loved ones in your life, and for simply being alive and well. Regardless of our sizes or how we look, we are incredibly fortunate.

· **Visualization**

Visualization is the technique of mentally rehearsing or forming a mental image of a desired result. Many Olympic and professional athletes use visualization to improve athletic performance. Dr. Kay Porter and Judy Foster, authors of the book *The Mental Athlete*, have suggested that "visualizing specific movements, performance techniques or personal endeavors creates neural patterns in the brain. The more one visualizes, the more ingrained these neural patterns become." We can, in fact, improve our physical world through *practice living* in our mental world. Explore this powerful tool.

Since the subconscious mind has a hard time distinguishing between what is visualized and what is actually experienced in the external world, visualization is an excellent tool for conscious change. When we are practicing a deep, rich, detailed visualization, we are able to create and experience our desired emotions. We send a powerful message to our subconscious mind, reinforcing the manifestation of our desires and goals.

Visualization takes many forms. Some people report that they experience a "feeling" more than seeing an actual image. Regardless of what style works for you, visualization is a great tool for focusing awareness and aligning our physical and mental energies with our spiritual purposes.

When I use visualizations, I imagine myself seated in a dark theater. As the velvet curtains draw, I watch the credits roll. I am the director and the producer of my mental movie, in which I also *happen* to be starring. Each time I visualize, the underlying theme is the same: to experience my perfect self, moving through life effortlessly, experiencing all that I desire. The plot line, location, and supporting characters may change, but the intent is the same. For just five minutes each morning I picture myself creating the ideal day.

Here is an example of a workday visualization: I am enjoying a relaxed morning. I take a refreshing shower, do a quick stretch, and drink a delicious fruit smoothie for breakfast. As my day at work unfolds, I picture myself being enthused, creative, and kind to those around me. I bring energy and laughter to others. I eat consciously at lunch and engage in positive conversation with friends. In the evening, I imagine heading out the door with my dog for a rejuvenating walk, appreciating all of the gorgeous scenery around me. Feeling content and relaxed, I picture myself connecting with a loved one, in whatever way I choose, maybe through a visit or a phone call. As I fall asleep, I express my gratitude for a full and satisfying life. Now that is a great day.

Visualizations are far from being hard work. Just think about how much fun it is to daydream. Visualizing is essentially just a focused daydream where you get to star in your own show, playing the main part in a script that you wrote! The ability for you to create an Oscar-winning mental image reinforces your deeply fulfilling, unfolding reality.

Try spending just a few minutes visualizing the experience of living in a fit, healthy body empowered by a peaceful mind. In detail, picture how the day will unfold. What do you choose to eat? How do you treat others? What do you think about? How do you deal with challenging issues? Visualize yourself turning down foods that don't serve you. Picture yourself lacing up your shoes and heading out the door for a walk. How do you feel? You can change the focus of your visualization whenever you like.

Using visualization plants the seeds of intention in our sub-conscious minds. We can experience all that we can imagine, and with every new day we are able to shape our realities by simply spending a little time playing out how we want our day to be. I often start my meditation with a powerful five-minute visualization.

·   **Create a library of positive, affirming, and spiritually inspired work**

Read. Study. Soak up some of the wonderful spiritual wisdom found in hundreds of popular books on the market today. Although most of the topics do not focus on losing weight, this important information builds our spiritual foundation, which is a fundamental factor in our weight loss success. Some of my favorite authors on the topic of spirituality and self-growth are Deepak Chopra, Wayne Dyer, Sarah Ban Breathnach, Ken Wilber, Marianne Williamson, Neil Donald Walsh, and the Dalai Lama's many books on Buddhism.

Use a daily book of affirmations. This is an effective and enjoyable way to bring attention back to our purpose, propelling us in the directions that we want to travel. Daily affirmations open our hearts and minds to the day that lies ahead.

Become familiar with the works of the great quantum physicists. Understanding scientific discoveries about the nature of physical reality is incredibly inspiring. Science is proving that matter and spirit actually stem from the same infinite field of energy. In its most rudimentary state, physical matter has been shown to be "nonmaterial," refuting the traditional view that *physical matter* and *spirit* arise from two independent entities. The scientists who write about the inseparability of physics and consciousness open our eyes to see spirit *in all material things*. We learn from these scientists that as humans, our two basic natures—the physical and the spiritual—are, in fact, inextricably linked. A good, nonthreatening place to start reading about this subject is Ken Wilber's book *Quantum Questions: Mystical Writings of the World's Great Physicists*. This is an anthology of non-technical excerpts taken from the mystical writings of great physicists such as Einstein, Heisenberg, Schrödinger, Jeans, Pauli, Eddington, Planck, and de Broglie (Shambhala Publications, 1985).

· **Commit to review and revise your soul food as needed**

I look over my soul-food recipe whenever I feel as if I am getting stagnant or bored. I revise my list every year. Do what suits you.

· **Use a journal**

In earlier generations it was common to keep a diary or personal journal. Today, few people do it, and very few recognize the value and astonishing power of writing down your thoughts and desires. Keeping a journal is a vital aspect of personal growth and self-understanding.

I have written in a journal, intermittently, for over eighteen years. Interestingly, I notice that I write most consistently when there are challenges in my life. It is not surprising that I wrote daily while recovering from my eating disorder. It provided me with great insight into my own soul.

I use my journal in many valuable ways:

To set the day's priority:

Each day, I plan to do just one loving thing for my body, mind, and spirit. For example:

"I will help someone today," or "I will get outside and walk for fifteen minutes," or "Just for today I will not judge my body." I don't feel overwhelmed when I take it one day at a time. I can do it for one day. I don't need to worry about the next ten years.

To make a gratitude list:

Each day I write down five things that I am grateful for—even if it means finding something small, like the radiant color of a flower, soaking in a hot lavender-scented bath, or peeking at the sliver of a disappearing moon. Everything counts. On some days this is my entire journal entry. I love looking back over the years remembering all of the little gems that brought me joy. When we focus on what we have versus what is missing, we shift our experience from the position of scarcity to one of abundance. The universe is complete—nothing is missing. Aligning ourselves with this abundance starts when we are grateful for what we already have. By recognizing our *wealth,* we open ourselves up to attract more and more. It's all about flow.

To help me recognize progress:

Unless we have a record, it can be difficult to recognize the small, positive changes taking place in our lives. It is so easy to forget how far we have actually come.

Just two months ago I went to the doctor to have a sore area in my breast examined. It was a benign fibrous lump. My doctor suggested giving up coffee as the caffeine might be contributing to the problem. The first few days were excruciating—I loved my morning cup of French Press. Today I drink decaf coffee, I don't miss caffeine, and my lump is entirely gone. When I review my journal, I remember how tough those first few days were. What a headache! My journal reminds me of my strength. I gave up coffee *in spite* of the discomfort. In addition, since I can revisit my unpleasant experience of caffeine withdrawal, I am less likely to go back to drinking coffee again.

One of the greatest rewards of keeping a journal comes from reading what we have written—months or years later—to recognize our valuable growth that goes unnoticed day to day.

To eliminate temptation:

When we write about our challenges and temptations with food, its power to control our actions diminishes. We are transferring this frustrated energy from our minds onto paper. When I am feeling stuck or indecisive about something I will take out a blank piece of paper and start to write. I *dump it all* onto that page and when I have vented my feelings satisfactorily, my mind is free. I find this incredibly helpful to eliminate temptations and restore inner balance.

To increase focus:

Using a journal clarifies my goals. As I write a few thoughts each day, my idea about what is important becomes much clearer. Keeping a journal helps me to discover what I really want to experience. Writing regularly simplifies my life—*I know my purpose*—and, therefore, staying on track is easier.

At the very least, a journal can help teach you important things about yourself and your relationship with food, body image, and weight. In whatever form it may take, use a journal to speak your truth. Without the safety of this space in which to grow, many personal discoveries would never have been born.

A Peaceful Mind Leads to a Lighter Body

When we learn to silence the incessant chatter of the mind and listen to the quiet voice inside, we begin to have clarity, there is calm, balance is restored, life seems more playful, we *experience* love, we heal. And yes, we begin to lose excess weight that no longer holds power over us. Old behaviors no longer serve a purpose as we have been blessed with a new level of consciousness to explore. *A peaceful mind is a powerful weight-loss tool.*

Incorporating these consciousness-raising tools into our lives can be effortless if we do it a little bit at a time. As you create your daily plan, simply choose one or two suggestions from this chapter and see how they work for you in your own life.

It's now time to . . .

Rip up your membership to the Diet Club once and for all!

Can we all agree that:

✓ Losing weight is not just about food and exercise.

✓ When we do the work—spiritually, emotionally, and physically—we will have all that we desire.

✓ Short-term restrictive diets are not an option.

✓ There is nothing to prove. We are here to fulfill the inherent desire of our spirits: to experience life fully by expressing and developing all that we are capable of being.

Read this affirming agreement. Sign it. Do what you need to do to say "yes" to a winning approach to long-term health and happiness.

Empowering Health Affirmation:

I will no longer subject myself to the punishment, impracticality, and deprivation of restrictive diets. I am choosing to commit to a holistic approach toward health that encompasses all of the spiritual, mental, and physical tools I need in order to experience optimal well-being and personal fulfillment.

I, _____, hereby commit to nurture my *whole* self.

Date: _____

CHAPTER ELEVEN

Creating a Masterpiece—One Ingredient at a Time

Today's preparation determines tomorrow's achievement.

B Y SELECTING INFORMATION from the work that you have already completed, I am going to help you build a simple daily plan that covers all of the necessary facets for achieving permanent weight loss and greater life fulfillment. By taking action daily—spiritually, mentally, and physically—we live our true essence, guaranteeing us the rich lives that we all desire.

Without direction, many of us never even get *started* on the journey toward greater freedom and personal empowerment. When we don't have a plan, we do what immediately "pays off." We may give in to immediate gratification, although it's only a temporary reward. By taking a little time each day to focus on the desires of our hearts, we have a reason to deny immediate gratification, emotional eating, and sedentary living. When we have a plan, we have purpose. It's the small daily steps we take that create an amazing life. Now *that's* rewarding.

Before we start to throw all of the ingredients into one big melting pot, review each question below to ensure that you are satisfied with your previously completed work.

❑ You have personally decided that changing your beliefs and lifestyle in order to lose weight is a worthy goal (Exercise 2, questions 1–3, page 40).

❑ You have pinpointed the positive emotions associated with being healthier and more fit by remembering or imagining how incredibly freeing it feels to live in this empowered state (Exercise 3, question 1, page 55).

❑ You have identified the emotions that you want to avoid by clearly stating examples of how you feel when you are not living an inspired life (Exercise 3, question 2, page 59).

❑ You have chosen to free yourself from the weight loss struggle (Exercise 3, question 3, page 61).

❑ You have created an extensive soul food list that nourishes your authentic self (Exercise 4, page 66).

Putting It All Together

The following outline is the basic framework for your recipe. Each essential component of the recipe has a daily action to fulfill. To give you a clear idea of how the daily plan works, I have used an example from my own recipe book. Refer to this example when writing your entries in the worksheet provided in the Appendix. You can get started today and, for future recipe worksheets, either photocopy the sample or draw up your own on a computer. Personalize it as you like.

The Empowering Health "Daily Recipe"
(An example from my journal)

Quote of the day:

On pages 163–168 you will find over three months' worth of inspirational quotes to get you started. Each morning choose one that you like and set the tone for your day.

"We are what we repeatedly do; Excellence, then, is not an act but a habit."

1. Spiritual/Inspirational:

Gratitude list
Big or small, jot down at least three things that you feel grateful for.

1. *The gorgeous walk yesterday with Justice in the canyon.
   It was so green and fresh—I loved it.*
2. *A surprise e-mail from my good friend, Jill, in Australia.
   She's pregnant!*
3. *Ashek, the owner of my favorite breakfast spot, told me
   that breakfast was "on the house" yesterday!*

Choose one or more of these consciousness-raising tools
daily:

☑ Visualization:
   *I will spend five minutes at the start of my meditation
   visualizing my "ideal self" experiencing a perfect day.*
❑ Yoga
❑ Journal
❑ Refrain from judging self or others
❑ Pray
☑ Meditate:
   I will meditate for thirty minutes before breakfast.
❑ Read spiritually based work or use a book of daily af-
   firmations
❑ Spend time in silence or in nature
❑ Other consciousness-expanding tools (see Chapter 10 or
   implement your own)

2. Motivational:

Each day ask yourself:

1. What do I want?

Look at your soul food. Look at your SMART goals. These are your desires. You don't have to write them down—just review your written goals.

2. Why do I want it?

What are the rewards of living on purpose? How will you feel if you don't pursue your desires? (Review your lists from Chapter 6.)

3. Physical:

In what small way can you contribute to your physical health and well-being today? (This can be anything, no matter how significant. For example: make a phone call inquiring about the walking group in your area, skip dessert, take a fitness class, do ten sit-ups, walk for fifteen minutes, stretch while you watch TV, *anything*. It all counts.)

1. Nutrition and eating:
   I will cook a nutritious meal tonight instead of eating out.
2. Activity:
   I will walk for fifteen minutes after dinner.

Pick just *one thing* from your soul food and implement it into your day.

3. Soul Food:

I will have a candle-lit bath with essential oils this evening.

Potential obstacles today:

As usual, I don't have any groceries in my fridge in order to cook dinner when I get home—the main reason why I usually eat out.

Troubleshooting obstacles:

Instead of stopping on the way home to buy a prepared meal, I will pick up fresh vegetables and halibut at the grocery store for tonight. In the future, stocking my kitchen with nutritious food just once or twice a week will ultimately save me more time and money than my usual eat-out plan, plus I will have tasty, nutritious options at home when hunger strikes.

The Evening Express:

Before you go to bed, summarize how your day progressed. How are you feeling now? This is your space to express yourself—no guidelines. From a brief sentence to a lengthy entry, write whatever you like.

Be blind to the small flaws, empower the positives of the day.

I had a great day today. I woke up with a sore back but I made the effort to stretch throughout the day and that made a big difference. In fact, I felt the best I had all day during my evening walk, which I extended from fifteen minutes to thirty-five. Instead of meditating before breakfast, I ended up doing twenty minutes during my relaxing candle-lit bath, finishing with a five-minute visualization of tomorrow's ideal day. I ate well today and although I ate a big portion at dinner, I prepared it at home—so good for me! A frustrating thing happened to me this afternoon. I lost a chunk of unsaved material on the computer. In the past, this would have ruined the rest of my day. Instead, I took a few deep breaths, closed my eyes, and focused on the bigger picture. Was it that big a deal? No. In fact when I rewrote the lost material, I think it turned out better anyway. Overall I had a very enjoyable day. I accomplished all of my goals in some form or another. I feel grateful for my full life. Good night. Love, Deb.

Remember . . .

When you are making your daily recipe, you don't *have* to do anything! Perhaps you just want to focus on one area of your plan for the first few weeks, and then add another component later. It's entirely up to you. In order to achieve long-term weight loss, you will ultimately want to include some form of daily action that feeds you spiritually, emotionally, and physically. Take your time. Confucius said, "It does not matter how slowly you go so long as you do not stop."

Just for Today

Abraham Lincoln said, "The best thing about the future is that it comes only one day at a time. So make the best of it today." This is so true; especially when it comes to weight loss. We need only focus our attention on the next sixteen hours. That's it. Although making this recipe may seem like a lot of work at first, within a few days it will take *only five minutes* to write down the day's priorities. The more often you do it, the easier it will be until one day, you will no longer need to make a daily plan. But until that moment comes . . .

Just for today can you connect with the intrinsic desires of your heart—commit to the health and well-being of your body, yet remain detached from the number on the scale?

Just for today are you willing to invest the time it takes to look at your life objectively and challenge your current beliefs?

Just for today are you committed to living a more authentic life—one that connects you to your true essence?

Just for today do you accept the physical importance of healthy eating and engaging in moderate activity?

And, lastly, *just for today* can you be grateful for your life, regardless of the size of your body?

These are tough questions; no doubt about it. We all fluctuate between "yes," "no," and "sometimes." Yet the more often we can *step up to the plate* and say "yes" to taking responsibility, and to acting passionately with regard to who we are, losing weight becomes integrated with all of the other joyous experiences going on in our lives.

Saying "yes" is a process that requires an ongoing commitment to honoring our *non-ego* self—the timeless, spiritual self that is inherent in every one of us. Each day that we nurture and honor our *whole* selves, we get closer to experiencing the effortlessness and beauty of who we really are. You have been given a blank canvas—the gift called life—already complete without a stroke of color. With love as your paintbrush, give back a masterpiece.

APPENDIX

Exercises

Exercise #1
Writing Your Story

I encourage you to take some time to write your own story. Feel free to use any format that you feel comfortable with. This exercise is for your eyes only, so try to be as thorough, honest, and reflective as you can. If you have a hard time getting started or get stuck along the way, use some of these questions to guide your writing:

- When did you first begin to have issues with food?
- When did you first start to gain excess weight?
- What was going on in your life?
- How did you feel about yourself?

- Are there any patterns in your story?
- What weight-loss methods have you tried?
- How did these different techniques make you feel?
- What have you learned?
- Where are you today?

_____

_____

_____

_____

_____

_____

_____

_____

_____

_____

_____

_____

_____

_____

_____

_____

_____

_____

_____

_____

_____

_____

_____

_____

_____

_____

_____

_____

_____

_____

_____

_____

_____

_____

_____

_____

_____

_____

_____

_____

_____

_____

_____

_____

_____

_____

_____

_____

Exercise #2

QUESTION ONE: Why do you want to lose weight?

Why is it important to you—or is it? Are you concerned about your health? Are you trying to make others happy? Do you want to look better in a bathing suit? What is your primary motivation? What do you think will happen in your life when you lose weight? Other than the size of your body, what will change? Whether you consider them silly or serious, list all of the reasons why you want to lose weight or improve your overall health and well-being.

_____

_____

_____

_____

_____

_____

_____

_____

_____

_____

_____

_____

_____

_____

_____

_____

QUESTION TWO: Are you willing to challenge yourself and work at your goal?

Making the commitment to improve our health takes effort. Change, for many of us, can bring up emotions that we may not feel comfortable experiencing. Are the reasons why you want to change important enough to you that you are willing to work at reaching your goal? Whether you are changing your physical lifestyle (activity level or eating habits) or altering ingrained beliefs about weight loss, are you willing, at times, to feel challenged? Are you willing to be courageous and have faith walking this new path in order to experience your true essence?

_____

_____

_____

_____

_____

_____

_____

_____

_____

_____

_____

_____

_____

_____

QUESTION THREE: *Are you willing to accept, love, and nurture your whole self—independent of weight loss?*

What actually makes a person lovable? Is it just their body? Beyond the physical, what is attractive about you? What do family, friends, and coworkers like about you? Do you think your attitude toward your own body is loving? Are you willing to change the way you see yourself?

Exercise #3

QUESTION ONE: *What does being fit and healthy feel like to you?*

Start by reflecting on the times in your life when you felt connected to your body—free to enjoy the pleasures of health and well-being—liberated from self-judgment. How did being healthy *feel*? What was it like to be in your body? How did health affect your mental and emotional experience?

_____

_____

_____

_____

_____

_____

_____

_____

_____

_____

_____

_____

_____

_____

_____

_____

QUESTION TWO: *What experiences or feelings emerge when you fail to take care of your health?*

_____

_____

_____

_____

_____

_____

_____

_____

_____

_____

_____

_____

_____

_____

_____

_____

_____

_____

_____

_____

_____

_____

_____

QUESTION THREE: Do you want to feel freedom?

What obstacles or actions are stopping you from experiencing your "healthy and fit" list right now? When you look at your list of "unhealthy" experiences, are you okay with feeling this way? Who or what is stopping you from feeling free? Are you content to continue living in this manner?

_____

_____

_____

_____

_____

_____

_____

_____

_____

_____

_____

_____

_____

_____

_____

_____

_____

_____

_____

_____

_____

Exercise #4
Soul Food

This exercise is intended to help you reconnect with the things that add joy and passion to your life. I have provided some brainstorming suggestions to help you get started.

- List the items or activities that make you feel cared for. (Some examples include: getting a massage, sharing your worries with a trusted loved one, going to bed early, getting a haircut, and so on.)

_____

_____

_____

_____

_____

_____

_____

_____

- What makes you laugh? What makes you feel silly and carefree? In whose company do you feel happy?

_____

_____

_____

_____

_____

_____

_____

_____

• How do you relax (by taking a bath, listening to music, meditating, watching your favorite show on TV, changing into your pajamas, playing with your kids, reading a book, going for a walk, catching up with friends, writing in your journal, and so on)?

_____

_____

_____

_____

_____

_____

_____

• What makes you feel attractive (living with confidence, dancing slowly, being witty, dressing up, and so on)?

_____

_____

_____

_____

_____

_____

• What do you do that contributes to a good day at work (getting organized, experiencing harmony with coworkers, taking moments out to decrease stress, finishing a project, bringing positive energy to others, and so on)?

_____

_____

_____

_____

_____

_____

_____

- Look around the surroundings in your home. What do you enjoy about your residence? How can you create more pleasure where you live? (Why don't you get rid of the junk and only keep items that you *love* or *use*? Give unused clothing and household items to the needy, place fresh flowers anywhere, light candles, paint, organize photos, rearrange a messy corner, diffuse essential oils throughout the house, clean out cupboards, hang a new item on the wall, and so on.)

_____

_____

_____

_____

_____

_____

- What are you interested in learning about (using a computer, investing, changing the oil in your car, meditating, traveling in Nepal, dancing, and so on)?

_____

_____

_____

_____

_____

_____

_____

- What do you want to improve or develop in yourself, your community, or the world?

_____

_____

_____

_____

_____

_____

- What do you enjoy doing with your partner, your friends, your parents, your children? How do you nurture your loved ones?

_____

_____

_____

_____

_____

_____

- Ultimately, what do you desire in your life?

_____

_____

_____

_____

_____

_____

_____

Exercise #5

Creating **SMART** Goals

1. Goal: _____

_____

SMART breakdown

Specific _____

Measurable _____

Adaptable _____

Realistic _____

Time frame _____

2. Goal: _____

_____

SMART breakdown

Specific _____

Measurable _____

Adaptable _____

Realistic _____

Time frame _____

3. Goal: _____

_____

SMART breakdown

Specific _____
Measurable _____
Adaptable _____
Realistic _____
Time frame _____

4. Goal: _____

_____

SMART breakdown

Specific _____
Measurable _____
Adaptable _____
Realistic _____
Time frame _____

Sample Daily Recipe

Date:

Quote of the day:

_____

_____

1. Spiritual/Inspirational:

Gratitude list
Big or small, jot down at least three things that you feel grateful for.

1. _____
2. _____
3. _____

Choose one or more of these consciousness-raising tools daily:

❏ Visualization
❏ Yoga
❏ Journal
❏ Refrain from judging self or others
❏ Pray
❏ Meditate
❏ Read spiritually based work or use a book of daily affirmations
❏ Spend time in silence or in nature

❑ Other consciousness expanding tools (see Chapter 10 or implement your own)

2. Motivational:

Each day ask yourself:

a. What do I want?

Look at your goals. Look at your soul food. What do you desire? You don't have to write them down—just review your written goals.

b. Why do I want it?

How do you feel living on purpose? How will you feel if you don't pursue your desires? Review your lists from Chapter Six.

3. Physical:

In what small way can I contribute to my physical health and well-being today?

a. Nutrition and eating:

_____

_____

b. Activity: _____

Pick just one thing from your soul food list and implement it into your day.

c. Soul Food: _____

Potential obstacles today: *Can you think of any difficulties that may arise?*

_____

_____

_____

Troubleshooting obstacles: *How can you be prepared for or plan around the potential problem?*

_____

_____

_____

The Evening Express:

In the evening, just before you go to sleep, reconnect with your purpose by reviewing the positive aspects of the day. This can be any length you like.

Be blind to the small flaws—empower the positives of the day.

_____

_____

_____

_____

_____

_____

_____

_____

_____

Daily Quotes for Inspired Living

Believe nothing, no matter where you read it, or who said it, no matter if I have said it, unless it agrees with your own reason and your own common sense.—*Buddha*

I wanted to change the world. But I have found that the only thing one can be sure of changing is oneself.—*Aldous Huxley*

The starting point of all achievement is desire. Keep this constantly in mind. Weak desire brings weak results, just as a small amount of fire makes a small amount of heat.—*Napoleon Hill*

Courage is resistance to fear, mastery of fear—not absence of fear.—*Mark Twain*

One person with a belief is equal to a force of ninety-nine with only interests.—*John Stuart Mill*

True enjoyment comes from activity of the mind and exercise of the body; the two are ever united.—*Baron Alexander von Humboldt* (German naturalist)

Do not wish to be anything but what you are and try to be that perfectly.—*Francis Sales*

He who has health, has hope; and he who has hope has everything.—*Arabian proverb*

The gem cannot be polished without friction, nor man perfected without trials.—*Chinese proverb*

There is nothing either good or bad, but thinking makes it so.—*William Shakespeare*

If you are pained by external things, it is not they that disturb you, but your own judgment of them. And it is in your power to wipe out that judgment now.—*Marcus Aurelius*

The ancestor of every action is a thought.—*Ralph Waldo Emerson*

Insanity is doing the same thing over and over, and expecting a different result.—*Albert Einstein*

All that we are is the result of what we have thought.—*Buddha*

Whatever you can do or dream, you can begin it. Boldness has genius, magic and power in it. Begin it now.—*Goethe*

Anything worth doing is worth doing poorly until you learn to do it well.—*Steve Brown*

People begin to grow the day they have the first real laugh at themselves.—*Anonymous*

There's no failure, only feedback.—*Anonymous*

If we all did the things we are capable of doing, we would literally astound ourselves.—*Thomas Edison*

Since I experience everything through my own body-mind, I create my own experience and I am responsible for what happens to me.—*Anonymous*

To choose one's attitude in any given set of circumstances is the last of the human freedoms—to choose one's own way.—*Viktor Frankl*

It's not what you are that holds you back, it's what you think you are not.—*Dennis Waitley*

If it's going to be, it's up to me.—*Robert Schuller*

Remember: you are the only person who thinks in your mind! You are the power and authority in your world.—*Louise Hay*

The best years of your life are the ones in which you decide your problems are your own. You don't blame them on your mother, the ecology or the President. You realize that you control your own destiny.—*Albert Ellis*

There's only one corner of the universe you can be certain of improving, and that's your own self.—*Aldous Huxley*

Failure is only the opportunity to more intelligently begin.— *Henry Ford*

You are your thoughts. Don't ever let anyone else have dominion over them.—*Shad Helmstetter*

You and I possess within ourselves, at every moment of our lives, under all circumstances, the power to transform the quality of our lives.—*Werner Erhard*

Things do not change, we change.—*Henry David Thoreau*

It is good to have an end to journey toward; but it is the journey that matters, in the end.—*Ursula K. Le Guin*

People with goals succeed because they know where they're going.—*Earl Nightingale*

You already have the precious mixture that will make you well. Use it.—*Rumi*

You don't just stumble into the future. You create your own future.—*Roger Smith*

Learn from the past in order to plan for the future, but live in the present.—*D. H. Everett*

Vision is the art of seeing the invisible.—*Jonathan Swift*

It is easier to act yourself into a new way of feeling, than think yourself into a new way of acting.—*Anonymous*

It is so critical to focus in life on what we want versus what we don't want.—*Tony Robbins*

Goals provide the energy source that powers our lives. One of the best ways we can get the most from the energy we have is to focus it. That is what goals can do for us; concentrate our energy.—*Dennis Waitley*

Every thought has a parallel action. Every prayer has a sound and physical form.—*Meditations of Rumi*

What the mind can conceive and believe, the mind can achieve.—*Napoleon Hill*

To succeed you need to find something to hold on to, something to motivate you, something to inspire you.—*Tony Dorsett*

Persistent people begin their success where others end in failure.—*Edward Eggleston*

Stay committed to your decisions, but stay flexible in your approach.—*Tony Robbins*

We are so vain that we even care for the opinion of those we don't care for.—*Maria von Ebner-Eschenbach*

No one can make you feel inferior without your consent.—*Eleanor Roosevelt*

The problem with the rat race is that even if you win, you're still a rat.—*Lily Tomlin*

It is not easy to find happiness in ourselves, yet it is impossible to find it elsewhere.—*Agnes Repplier*

Advice is what we ask for when we already know the answer but wish we didn't.—*Erica Jong*

If the world were a logical place, men would ride sidesaddle.—*Rita Mae Brown*

Nothing seems so tragic to one who is old as the death of one who is young, and this alone proves that life is a good thing.—*Zoe Atkins*

Learn to get in touch with the silence within yourself, and know that everything in life has purpose. There are no mistakes, no coincidences, all events are blessings given to us to learn from.—*Elisabeth Kübler-Ross*

Resolve to be thyself; and know, that he who finds himself, loses his misery.—*Matthew Arnold*

The mystery of life is not a problem to be solved, but is a reality to be experienced.—*J. J. Van der Leeuw*

You cannot teach a man anything; you can only help him find it within himself.—*Galileo*

When you sit with a nice girl for two hours, you think it's only a minute. But when you sit on a hot stove for a minute, you think it's two hours. That's relativity.—*Albert Einstein*

Two men look out through the same bars; one sees the mud and one sees the stars.—*Frederick Langbridge*

A person will be just about as happy as they make their minds up to be.—*Abraham Lincoln*

Reflect upon your present blessings, of which every man has plenty; not on your past misfortunes, of which all men have some.—*Charles Dickens*

Liberty of thought is the life of the soul.—*Voltaire*

Procrastinating is the art of keeping up with yesterday.—*Don Marquis*

Your mind will give back exactly what you put into it.—*Anonymous*

Love is everything. It is the key to life, and its influences are those that move the world.—*Ralph Waldo Trine*

First keep the peace within yourself, then you can also bring peace to others.—*Thomas à Kempis*

RESOURCES

Web Sites

The following web sites have given me hours of wonderful reading, learning, and inspiration. Browse for yourself and please share them with those who you feel may benefit.

Deepak Chopra and the Chopra Center for Well Being:

Deepak Chopra's web site is filled with wonderful discussions, articles, and a wealth of spiritual inspiration. I check in regularly to the *Ask Deepak* discussion boards or to browse the *Wisdom Within* link. www.chopra.com

For a daily dose of motivation:
www.greatday.com

HALO Radio:

HALO Radio is a syndicated radio program in the United States and Canada, covering topics from Health, Anti-aging, Lifestyle, and alternate Options (HALO). Halo features notable luminaries from the health and wellness field. www.halo-on-air.com

Meditation made easy:

This user-friendly site was created to provide clear, straightforward meditation instruction to people anywhere on the planet. Make sure to check out the "links room" at the bottom of the home page. It is one of the most comprehensive and varied lists of links that I have found on the net—far too long to list here. This site has everything your soul needs! www.meditation center.com

National Women's Health Information Center:

This web site and toll-free call center was created to provide free, reliable health information for women everywhere. www. 4woman.gov

Quotes to inspire and motivate:

Add some of these gems to your daily recipe. www.motivational quotes.com

Run for your lives!

Everything a woman needs to know about running, from getting started, women's concerns, body and health issues, and much more. www.womens-running.com

Vegetarian Resource Group:

For all of your vegetarian needs. Recipes, nutritional information and even a vegetarian game!
www.vrg.org

ORGANIZATIONS

The following is a list of organizations that can provide assistance, information, or services for various areas of interest. Please be aware that addresses and telephone numbers are subject to change.

American Council on Exercise (ACE)
4851 Paramount Drive
San Diego, California 92123
(858) 279-8227 Toll Free 800-825-3636
www.acefitness.org

Alliance for Eating Disorders Awareness
The Alliance is a nonprofit organization dedicated to the public education and awareness of eating disorders. For more information, contact The Alliance at (561) 841-0900 or www.eating disorderinfo.org

American Dietetic Association (ADA)
The ADA is the nation's largest organization of food and nutrition professionals whose web site provides a wealth of nutrition information ranging from news releases and consumer tips to nutrition fact sheets and the Good Nutrition Reading List. Use the "Find a Dietitian" feature on ADA's web site.
www.eatright.org

National Eating Disorders Association (NEDA)
NEDA's mission is to eliminate eating disorders and body dissatisfaction through prevention efforts, education, referral and
support services, advocacy, training, and research.
603 Stewart Street, Suite 803, Seattle, WA 98101
Information and Referral Help Line 1-800-931-2237
www.nationaleatingdisorders.org

National Center for Overcoming Overeating
P.O. Box 1257
Old Chelsea Station
New York, NY 10113
212-875-0442

ABOUT THE AUTHOR

Deborah Low's passion and commitment to strive for and learn about healthy living has been prevalent throughout much of her thirty years, though there were times when she wandered from the *true source of wellness*.

As a healthy fourteen-year-old girl she began the all-too-common descent into anorexia. By sixteen she was an accredited fitness instructor, and by her late teens she was a full-blown bulimic.

When it was as though life had lost all bearing, something happened while she was in her second year of university. Deborah began to get better. She had been introduced to the teachings of the Behaviorists and began applying their work to her own shaky model of personal well-being. Using Behavior Modification, in particular, she found resounding effects for both herself and the women she trained. Without knowing it, she was discovering the mind's inherent motivators with regards to health. It is here, in the psychological domain, where Deborah's own self-destructive behavior began to slowly diminish; her bulimia, indeed, was getting better.

The years following university took her further into the psychological teachings. Reading and studying, reworking her recipe, formulating new ideas, by age twenty-three she was standing somewhat on her own but still vulnerable. Most days she felt bothered, but okay. Her mind and body craved more; and here the real studies began.

Deborah began to compose a spiritual framework through which she could reconnect to her overall sense of self, using daily meditation, research, and reading. Deborah infused her spiritual understandings into the world of health and fitness. Over the years she formulated a scratch-book of ideas and notes and quotes which she would read through on the tough days. She cut out positive, inspiring photos from magazines to remind her of what to be grateful for. She scribbled down lists and lists of rainswept words to quench her silent thirst. Without knowing it, she had begun to discover what was with her all along. She began to hear her inner voice speaking in encouraging whispers. She began to feel the world around her on the hairs of her skin. For the first time in her life she understood that within her were all the essential ingredients to create a bountiful life.

Today, Deborah lives an inspiring life that nine years earlier was, in her words, "just okay." Deborah intends to share her joy with other women. To share her love. Share her freedom. Share her recipe for health.

Deborah holds a Bachelor of Arts degree from the University of Victoria in Psychology/Sociology and a Kinesiology certificate from Simon Fraser University. She is an accredited A.C.E. Certified Lifestyle and Weight Management Consultant working in community recreation as a Fitness, Health, and Wellness Programmer. Over the last few years, Deborah has spent several weeks at the Chopra Center for Well Being as both volunteer and course participant. She lives in Vancouver, Canada, and continues to write about inspiring health in mind, body, and spirit.

Deborah would be delighted to hear from you. She can be reached by e-mail at deborah@deborahlow.com. To sign up for her free newsletter, please visit her web site at www.deborahlow.com.